CW01583174

ENCYCLOPAEDIA OF INDIAN MEDICINE

VOLUME ONE
HISTORICAL PERSPECTIVE

Editor
Vidyalankara Prof. S.K. RAMACHANDRA RAO
President,Ayurveda Academy, Bangalore

POPULAR PRAKASHAN MUMBAI

On behalf of
Dr. V. PARAMESHVARA CHARITABLE TRUST, Bangalore

ENCYCLOPAEDIA
OF
INDIAN MEDICINE PROJECT

VOLUME ONE

Sponsored by
Dr. V. P. Parameshvara Charitable Trust
Bangalore

Chairman
Dr. V. Parameshvara
M.B.B.S.,F.R.C.P. (London), F.A.C.C.,F.C.C.P.,F.I.C.A.,
F.I.S.E.,F.A.I.I.D.,M.S.A.,F.I.A.M.S.,F.I.C.N.

Editor
Vidyalankara Prof. S. K. Ramachandra Rao
President, Ayurveda Academy, Bangalore

© Dr. PARAMESHVARA CHARITABLE TRUST,
Bangalore

First published 1985
First Reprint 1998
Second Reprint 2005
Third Reprint 2012
ISBN : 81-7154-255-7

(3302)

Printed in India by :
Saurabh Printers Pvt. Ltd.
Noida

Published by RAMDAS BHATKAL for
Popular Prakashan Pvt. Ltd.
35-C Pandit Madan Mohan Malaviya Marg,
Tardeo, Mumbai-400 034

ENCYCLOPAEDIA
OF
INDIAN MEDICINE

लोकाः समस्ताः
सुखिनो भवन्तु ॥

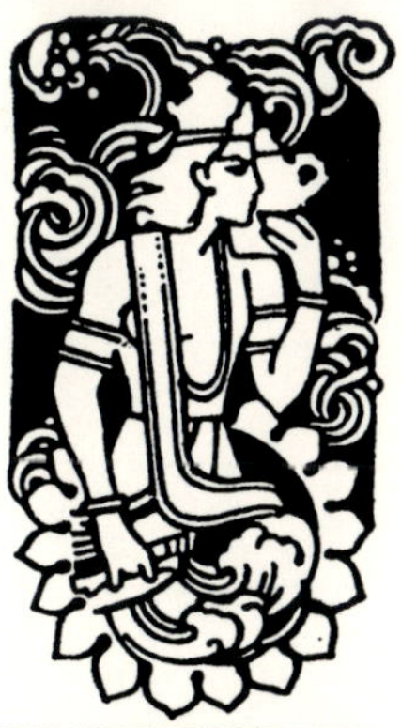

SRI DHANVANTARI

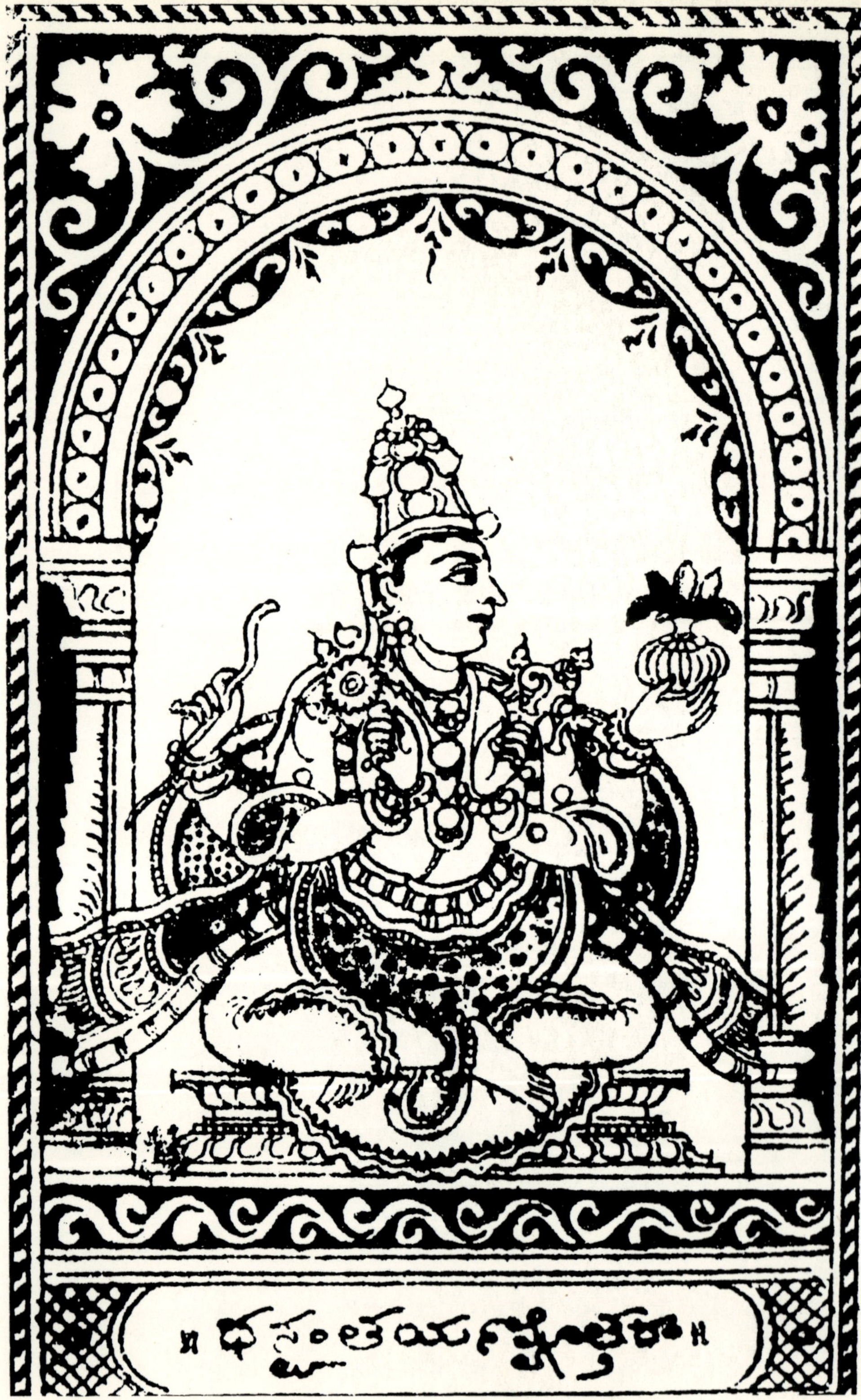

DHANVANTARI: from a painting got made by the late Mahārāja of Mysore, Krishnarāja Wodeyar III, for inclusion in his lithographic book Devatā-nāma-kusumāñjali.

PREFACE

Indian religions are well known in the world. The philosophical systems that emerged on the Indian soil have also engaged the attention of scholars all over the world. India's achievements in the field of science and technology have also been recognised. However, the fact that India developed a system of medicine, thousands of years ago, has not received wide coverage in the world. And that the system thus developed is still prevalent among the masses of India is likewise not generally known, even to historians of medicine.

There are manifold reasons for this general ignorance of Indian medicine among historians of medicine, medical practitioners outside the country and intelligentsia interested in the problems of health and disease. One is, absence of authoritative and well documented publications in English by Indians, dealing with this branch of medicine. The European indologists who have taken an interest in Indian medicine and have written on the subject do not seem to carry much credibility, because they are alien to the traditional details which are indispensable to the understanding of the spirit, outlook and value of Indian medicine. The literature available on this topic written in the traditional style of Indian languages have proved to be enigmatic to the modern reader. A great need is, therefore, felt for an authentic publication which communicates to the modern mind the traditional wisdom of India concerning medical practice.

The Encyclopaedia of Indian Medicine in six volumes has been planned to fulfil this need. The first volume provides the historical perspective as well as acquaintance with the medical literature in India. The volume has been prepared by Vidyalankara Prof. S.K. Ramachandra Rao, who hails from a family of traditional physicians and is the President of the Ayurveda Academy, Bangalore. Besides being a Sanskrit scholar and well versed in Ayurveda, he has also been a scientific worker, having headed the department of Clinical Psychology at the National Institute of Mental Health and Neurosciences, Bangalore (with which he is still associated as consultant to the Ayurvedic Research Unit).

The volume will be followed in due course by other volumes dealing with the basic ideas; methods of clinical investigation, therapeutic procedures, pharmaceutical practices and materia medica of Indian medicine. It is hoped that a comprehensive and factual knowledge of Indian medicine will be available to the world when the series is completed.

Bangalore
October 4, 1984

V. PARAMESHVARA
Chairman

INTRODUCTION

Indigenous medical wisdom in India known as Ayurveda goes back to a hoary past. Even in the early strands of the Vedic corpus belonging to a period several centuries prior to the Christian era, we find references not only to medical practice but to elaborate medical theories. Medical wisdom in India was systematized at a slightly later period, and a remarkably rich medical literature has grown up since those days. Medical practice based on this systematization has continued to our own day, despite the growing popularity of Western medical practice.

Indian medical wisdom has unfortunately been confined to India; and the West is largely ignorant of it. Even in India, the traditional medical practice seems to be losing contact with the system as it was crystallized over two thousand years ago. This is so because much of the early and core medical literature, which is in Sanskrit, is still in manuscripts, hidden away in libraries and private collections; only a few major texts like Charaka's *saṁhita,* Suśruta's *Saṁhita* and Vāgbhaṭa's *Sangraha* and *Hṛdaya* have been printed and translated into English. The influence of the philosophical systems, especially of Sāṁkhya and Nyāya-Vaiśeshika, on medical thought in India has not been sufficiently appreciated. The generation of practising physicians who are also scholarly has almost disappeared. Thus the authentic tradition of Indian medical thought has not yet been presented to the modern mind. The medical world at large is almost entirely ignorant of the relevance or the value of Ayurveda.

The present series of volumes constituting *The Encyclopaedia of Indian Medicine* is an attempt to present in a manner that would appeal to the modern mind the theoretical and practical issues as was formulated in Ayurveda several centuries ago. In so doing, we have relied entirely on original texts, which constitute the nucleus of Ayurveda, and on the commentarial literature thereupon, and have attempted to reconstruct the authentic perspective of Ayurveda The following volumes have been planned and are under preparation:

Volume I Historical Perspective
Volume II Conceptual
Volume III Clinical Examination, diagnosis and methods of Treatment
Volume IV Diseases; Drugs and their preparations
Volume V Materia Medica (in two parts)
Volume VI Folk Medicine

The first volume is now being published. It traces the development of medical thought through the ages and provides information about all the important medical authors and about their works available in print or in manuscripts; and content analyses of the more important works have been given, based on the first-hand study of the original texts. The purpose is to present a comprehensive picture of medical literature that is extant in the country. To facilitate comparative study, allied Asian systems of medicine (e.g. Arabian, Chinese, Tibetan, Yunani) have also been noticed.

It has been kept in mind by those who are involved in this Project that the purpose of any encyclopaedia is not only to provide information but to relate it. The entries are designed to introduce the reader to the basic principles guiding Indian medicine in the context of the country's geography, history and culture. Care has been taken to present the details objectively, and in accordance with the traditional framework. We have refrained from taking sides in the controversy regarding the relative merits of the different systems of medicine.

While the present Encyclopaedia is ultimately based on the original texts, commentaries and annotations in Sanskrit, a large number of works on Ayurveda written and published in English and in some of the Indian languages (Hindi, Kannada, Telugu and Tamil) have been consulted, as also many elderly specialists in this system of medicine. We are indebted to all these authors and scholars. But the formulation of the concepts and their applications have uniformly been made in accordance with the original textual tradition disregarding later revisions, evaluations and amendments.

The enlightened interest of the eminent Cardiologist of Bangalore, Dr. V. Parameshvara has originated this project, and has been sustaining it. Being himself a physician trained in the best traditions of modern medicine, he is interested in the world getting acquainted with the contributions of traditional medicine in India so that there could be greater benefit to mankind.

Bangalore S.K. RAMACHANDRA RAO
October 4, 1984 *Editor*

CONTENTS

LIST OF ILLUSTRATIONS

ABBREVIATIONS & MAJOR REFERENCES

AD	Aruna-datta (author of SaSu)
AE	Āyurvedic Encyclopaedia, A. Lakshmipathi, Madras 1959, in 2 Vol.
AHr	Ashtāṅga-hṛdaya (Vāgbhaṭa, ed. A. M. Kunte, NS, Bombay, 1891)
ARH	Āyurveda-rasāyana (Hemādri on AHr)
AS	Ashtāṅga-saṁgraha (Vāgbhaṭa, ed. Atrideva Gupta, NS, Bombay, 1951, with Hindi tr.)
ASM	Āyurvedic System of Medicine, (Nāgendra Nāth Sengupta, Calcutta, 1919)
ASS	Ānandāśrama Sanskrit Series, Puṇe.
AV	Āyurveda-vijñānam (Vinodalāl Sengupta, Calcutta 1916 and 1928, in 2 vol.)
AVV	Āyurveda-vyadhi-vijñānam
B	Baidyanātha Āyurveda Bhavan, Nāgpur,
BNR	Bṛhan-nighaṇṭu-ratnākara (Bombay, 1891)
BP	Bhāva-prakāśa (Bhāvamiśra)
BPN	Bhāva-prakāśa-nighaṇṭu.
BR	Bhaishajya-ratnāvalī (ed. Govindadāsa, Calcutta, 1893)
BS	Bhela-saṁhitā (Bhela, ed. Calcutta Univ., 1921)
BSR	Basava-rājīyam (Basava-rāja, Madras, 1951 in Telugu ch.)
BYT	Bṛhad-yoga-taraṅgiṇī (Trimalla-bhaṭṭa)
C	Chowkhamba Series, Vārāṇasī.
Chkp	Chakrapapāṇi-datta (comm. on CS)
CMA	Clinical Methods in Ayurveda (Śrīkaṇṭha-mūrthy, C, Vārāṇasī, 1983)
CS	Charaka-saṁhitā (ed. Yādavji Trikumji Āchārya, NS Bombay, 1941)
CSS	Chikitsā-sāra-samgraha (Vangasena, Calcutta, 1884)
DGV	Dravya-guṇa-vijñāna (P.V. Sharma, C, Vārāṇasī, 1981, in Hindi, in 5 vol.)
DGVY	Dravya-guṇa-vijñānam (Yādavji Trikumji Āchārya, Nagpur, 1953)
DMA	Digestion and Metabolism in Ayurveda (Dwārakānāth, C, Calcutta, 1967)
DN	Dhanvantari-nighaṇṭu (ASS, Puṇe, 1927, includes RN)
GnS	Gaṇa-nāth Sen
GN	Gada-nigraha (Sodhala, Bombay 1911 and 1915)
HIM	History of Indian Medicine (Girīndranāth Mukhopādhyāya, Calcutta, 1923-26, in 3 vol.)
HIP	A History of Indian Philosophy (Surendranāth Dasgupta, Cambridge Univ. Press. Vol II, 1952)
HO	Osteology (Hoernle, Oxford, 1907)
HS	Hārīta-saṁhitā (Calcutta, 1887)

IMM	Indian Materia Medica (K. M. Nāḍkarṇi, Popular Prakashan, Bombay, Revised and enlarged, 1976, in 2 vol.)
JIM	Indian Medicine (Julius Jolly, translated from German into English, Kāshīkar, Puṇe, 1951)
KK	Kalyāṇa-kāraka (Ugrāditya, Sholāpur, 1940)
KS	Kāśyapa-saṁhitā (ed. Yādavji Trikumji Āchārya, NS, Bombay, 1938)
MK	Madhu-kosha (Vijaya-rakshita, Calcutta, 1876)
MMH	Materia Medica of the Hindus (Uday Chand Dutt, Calcutta, 1922)
MN	Mādhava-nidāna (Mādhavakara, ed. Yādavji Trikumji Āchārya, NS, Bombay, 1884)
MPN	Madana-pāla-nighaṇṭu (Madana-pāla)
NiS	Nibandha-saṁgraha (Ḍalhana, on SS, NS, Bombay, 1915)
NS	Nirṇayā-sāgar Press, Bombay.
PRM	Paryāya-ratna-mālā (Mādhava, Paṭṇā, 1946)
PS	Pratyaksha-śārīram (Gaṇanāth Sen, Calcutta, 1913)
PSH	Positive Sciences of Ancient Hindus (Brajendra Nāth Seal, New edition, Motilāl Banārsidāss, 1958)
PSS	Pārishadyam Śabdārtha-śārīram (B, Nāgpur, 1964)
RM	Rasendra-maṅgala (Nāgārjuna?, Goṇḍāl, 1924)
RN	Rāja-nighaṇṭu (Abhidhāna-chintāmaṇi, ASS, Puṇe)
RRS	Rasa-ratna-samucchaya (Nityanātha, ASS, Puṇe, 1890)
RV	ṚgVeda
RVS	Rasa-vaiśeshika-sūtra (Nāgārjuna?, Trivandrum, 1928, with the comm. of Narasiṁha)
SaS	Śārṅgadhara-saṁhitā (litho., Bombay, Śaka 1799 with Marāṭhī trans)
SaSu	Sarvāṅga-sundara (Aruṇa-datta on AHr, Bombay, 1889)
Sds	Śiva-dāsa-sena
SdN	Soḍhala-nighaṇṭu (Soḍhala, BORI, Baroda; Puṇe 1972)
SHM	A History of Medicine (H. Sigerist, Oxford, 1951-1961, in 2 vol.)
SIH	Surgical Instruments of the Hindus (Girīndra Nāth Mukhopādhyāya, Calcutta Univ., 1913-1914)
SK	Sāṁkhya-kārikā (Īśvara-kṛshṇa)
SKD	Śabda-kalpa-druma (Rājā Rādhākānta Deb, C, Vārāṇasī, 3rd ed., 1967, in 5 parts)
SM	Siddha-mantra (Keśava, ed. Śankar Dāji Śāstrī, Bombay, 1897)
SMP	Siddha-mantra-prakāśa (Vopadeva, Madras, 1860)
SN	Śāligrāma-nighaṇṭu (Lālā Śāligrām, Vārāṇasī, 1891)
SS	Suśruta-saṁhitā (Suśruta, ed. Yādavji Trikumji Āchārya, NS, Bombay, 1915)
SSS	Suśruta-samhitā: A Scientific Synopsis (P. Ray et al., Indian National Science Academy, New Delhi 1980)
sth.	sthāna
su.	sūtra
SY	Siddha-yoga (Vṛnda, Puṇe, 1894)
VGP	Vastu-guṇa-prakāśikā (Vāsudeva-śāstri, Rājamahendravaram, 1938, in Telugu)
VJ	Vaidya-jīvana (Lolaṁba-rāja, Bangalore, 1923, in Kannaḍa ch.)
VRM	Vaidyaka-ratna-mālā (MSS copy)
VSS	Vaidyaka-śabda-sindhu (Umesh Chandra Gupta, Calcutta, 1894)
VSSK	Vaidya-sāra-saṁgraha (Bangalore, 1882, in Kannaḍa ch.)
VyK	Vyākhyā-kaumudi (MSS copy)
Vymk	Vyākhyā-madhu-kosha (MSS copy)
YR	Yoga-ratnākara (ASS, Puṇe, 1889; Mysore, 1899 in Kannaḍa ch., with Kannaḍa and Telugu trans.)
YV	Yajurveda
ZHM	Hindu Medicine (H. Zimmer, Baltimore, 1948)

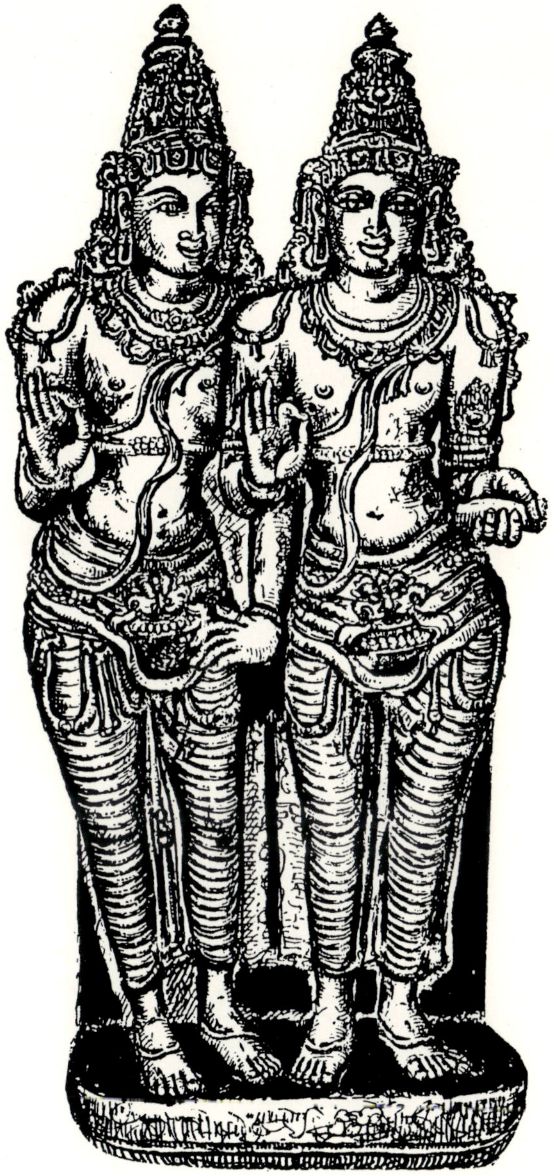

AŚVINĪ-DEVAS: adopted from Śilpi's sketch from a sculpture in the temple at Chidambaram in South India, originally made for the Tamil periodical *Ānandavikaṭan*.

Galaxy of Indian Men of Medicine

लोकाः समस्ताः
सुखिनो भवन्तु ॥

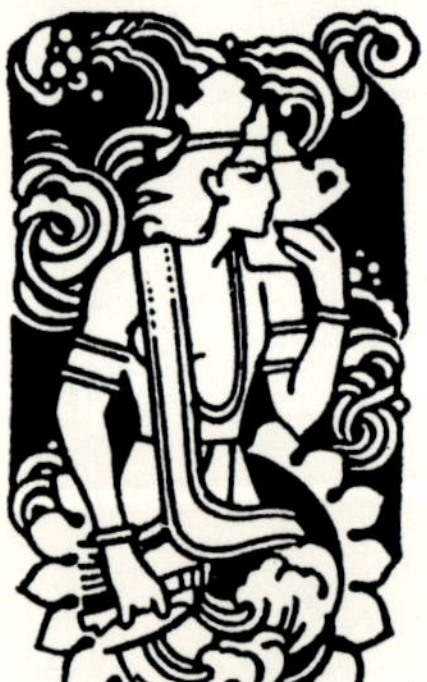

SRI DHANVANTARI

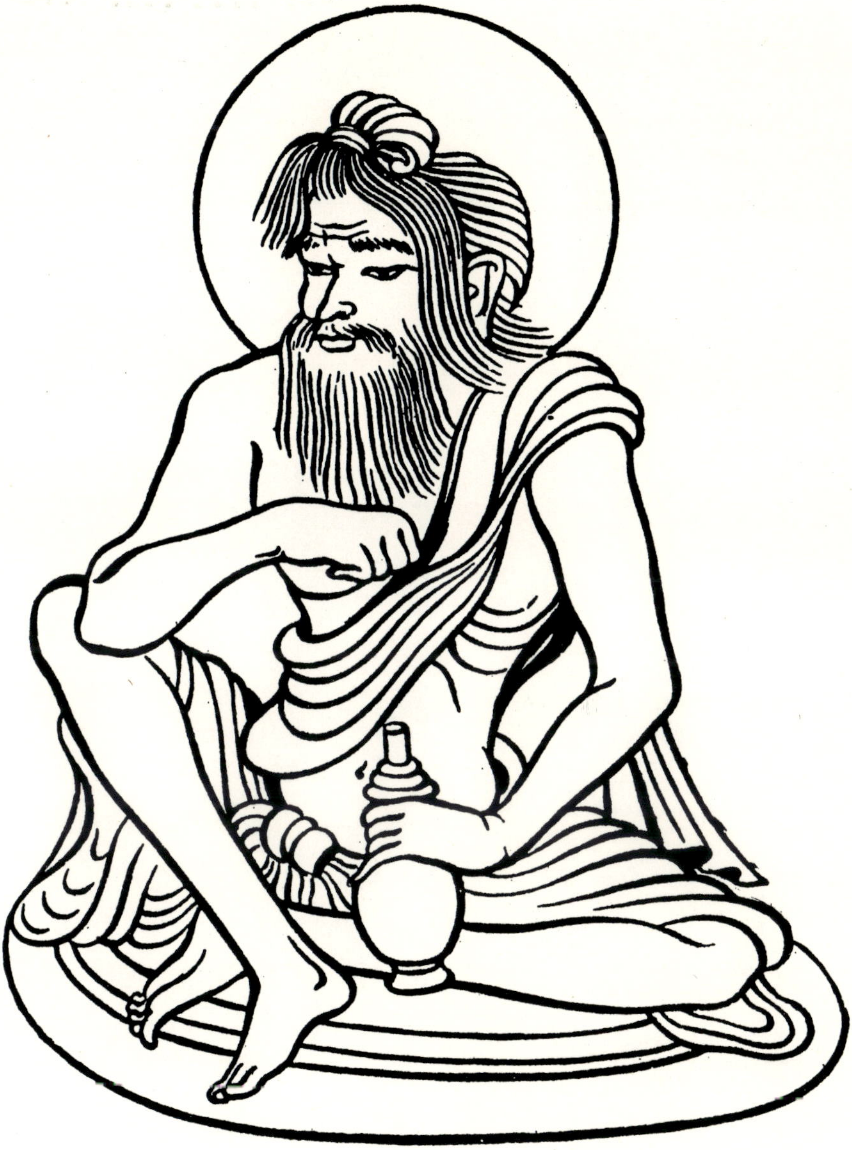

ĀTREYA: from a Mahāyāna manuscript (reproduced in Hobogirin's *Japanese-Chinese Dictionary of Buddhist Terms*), appearing as Plate III in Radha Kumud Mookerji's *Ancient Indian Education*, Motilal Banarsidass, Delhi, 1969.

PĀTAÑJALI: who is credited with having redacted *Charaka-Saṁhitā: adapted from Śilpi's a sketch of a sculptural representation in Chidambaram temple.*

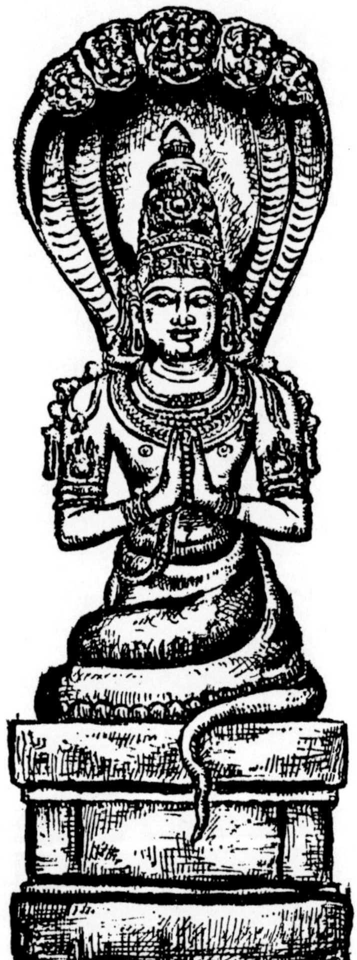

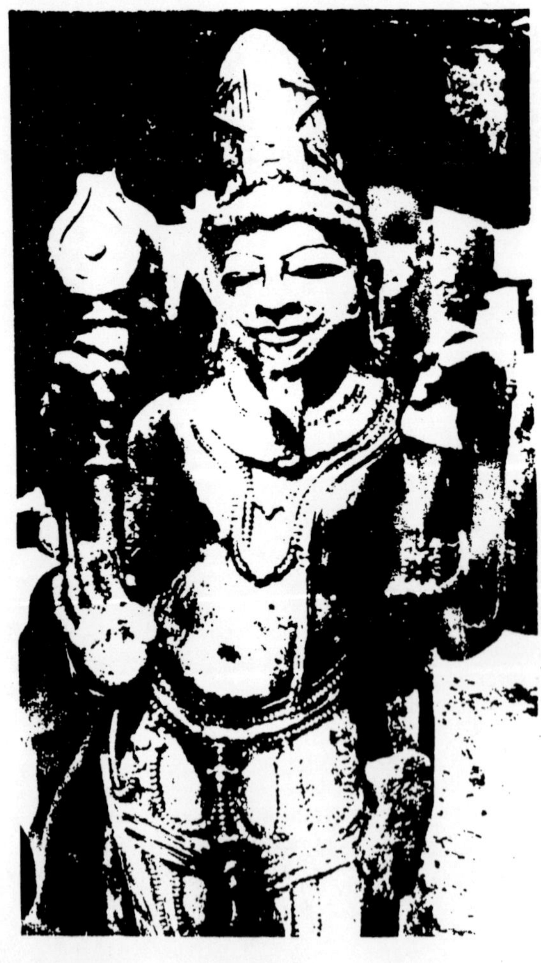

BRAHMA: A sculpture from Khajuraho Temple.

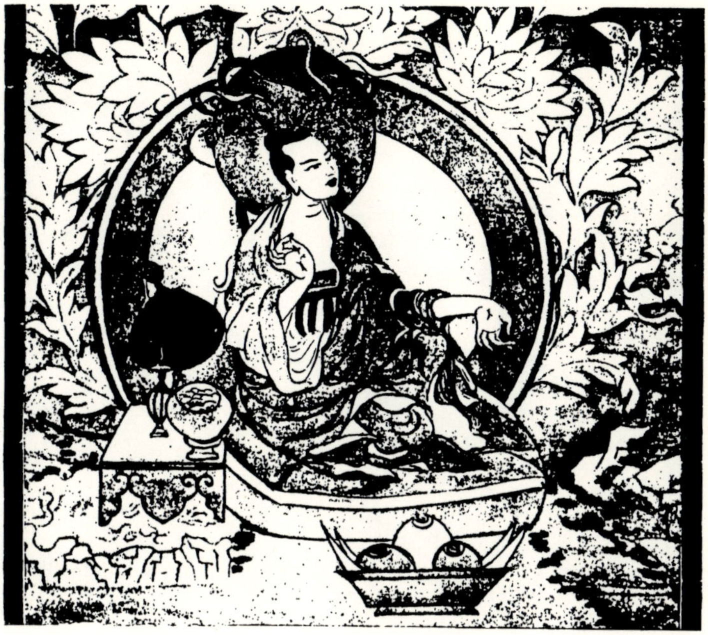

NĀGĀRJUNA: from a Tibetan scroll-painting.

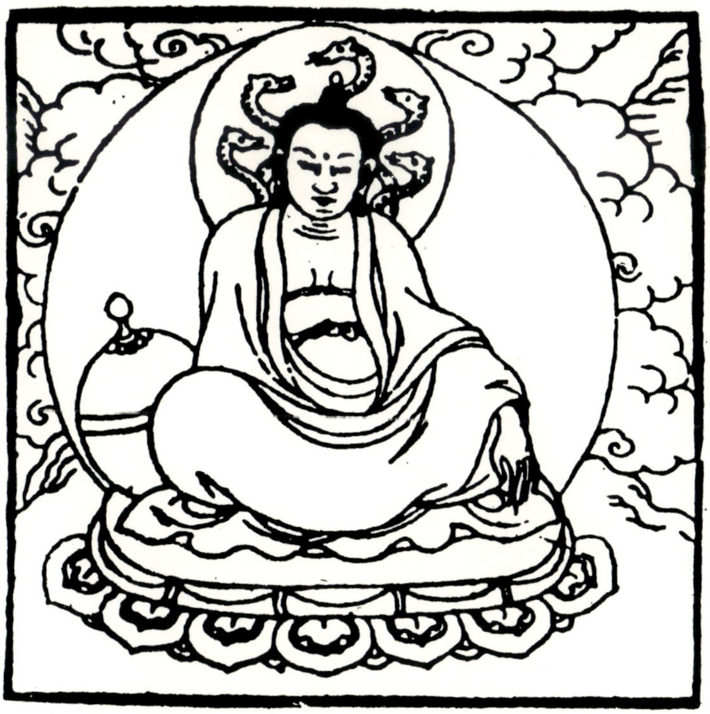

NĀGĀRJUNA: from a Tibetan manuscript, xylograph.

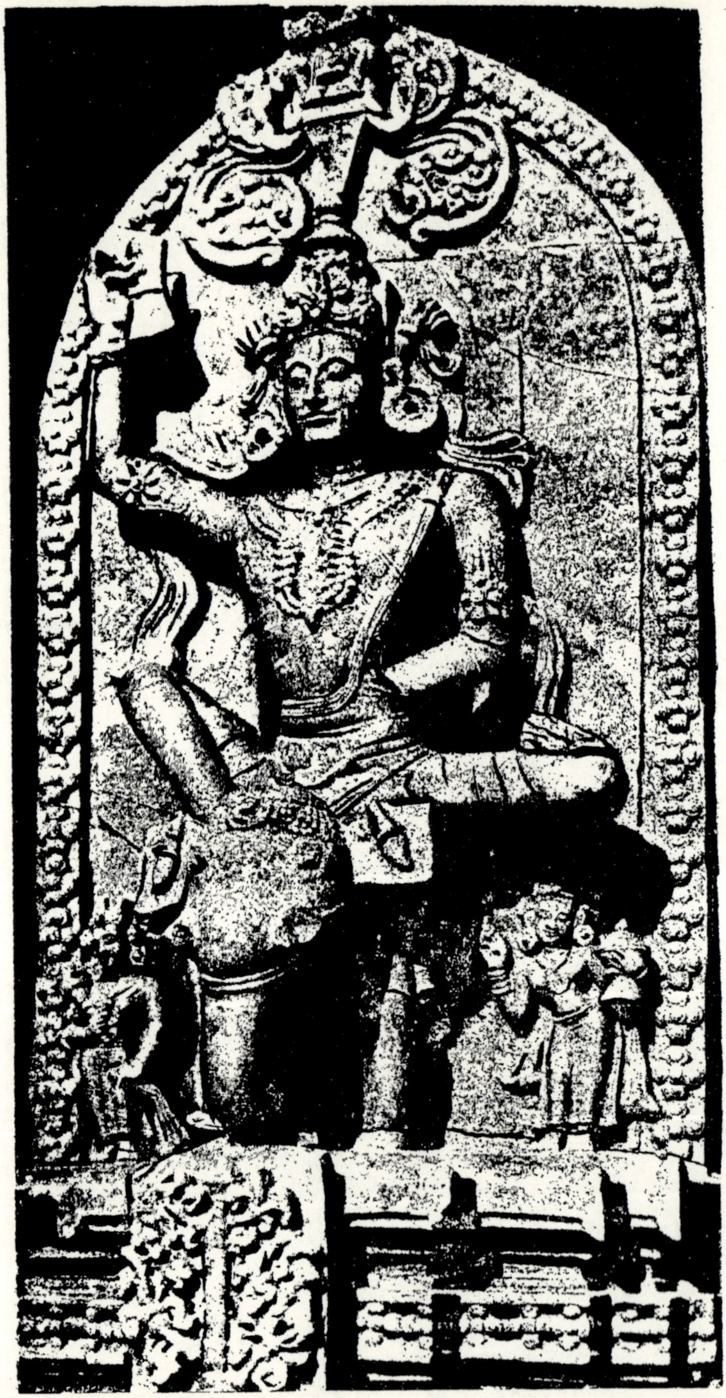

INDRA: from a sculptured panel in the Malinithan temple, Assam, reproduced in A. Bhattacharjee's *Icons and Sculptures of Early and Medieval Assam*, Inter-India Publications, Delhi, 1978.

SŪRYA: adapted from a Śilpi's sketch of a sculpture in Chidambaram temple in South India, originally made for the Tamil periodical, *Ānandavikatan*.

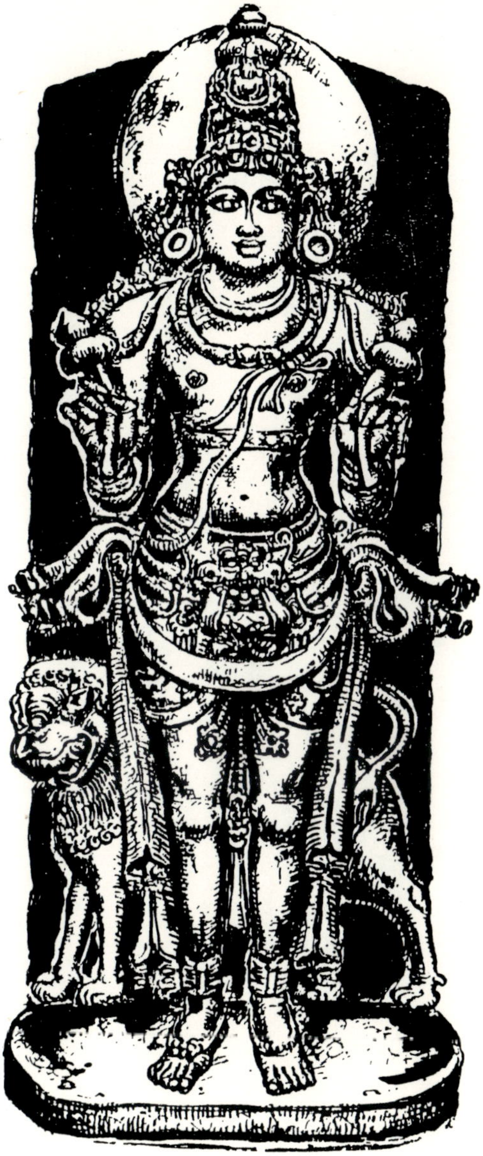

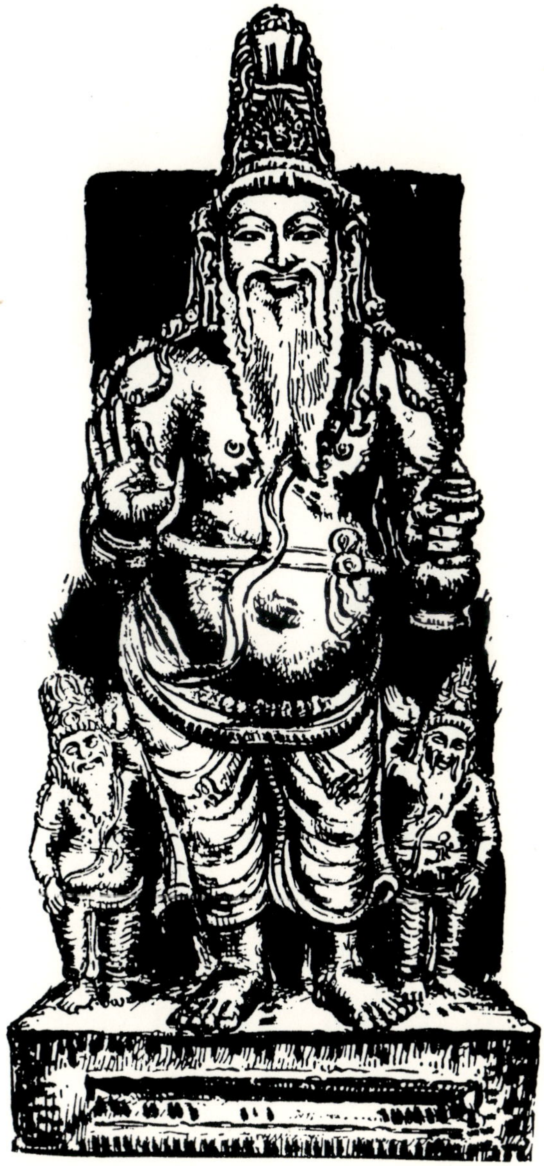

The Sage AGASTYA: adapted from Śilpi's sketch of a sculpture in the Chidambaram temple (South India), originally reproduced in the Tamil periodical *Āndavikatan*.

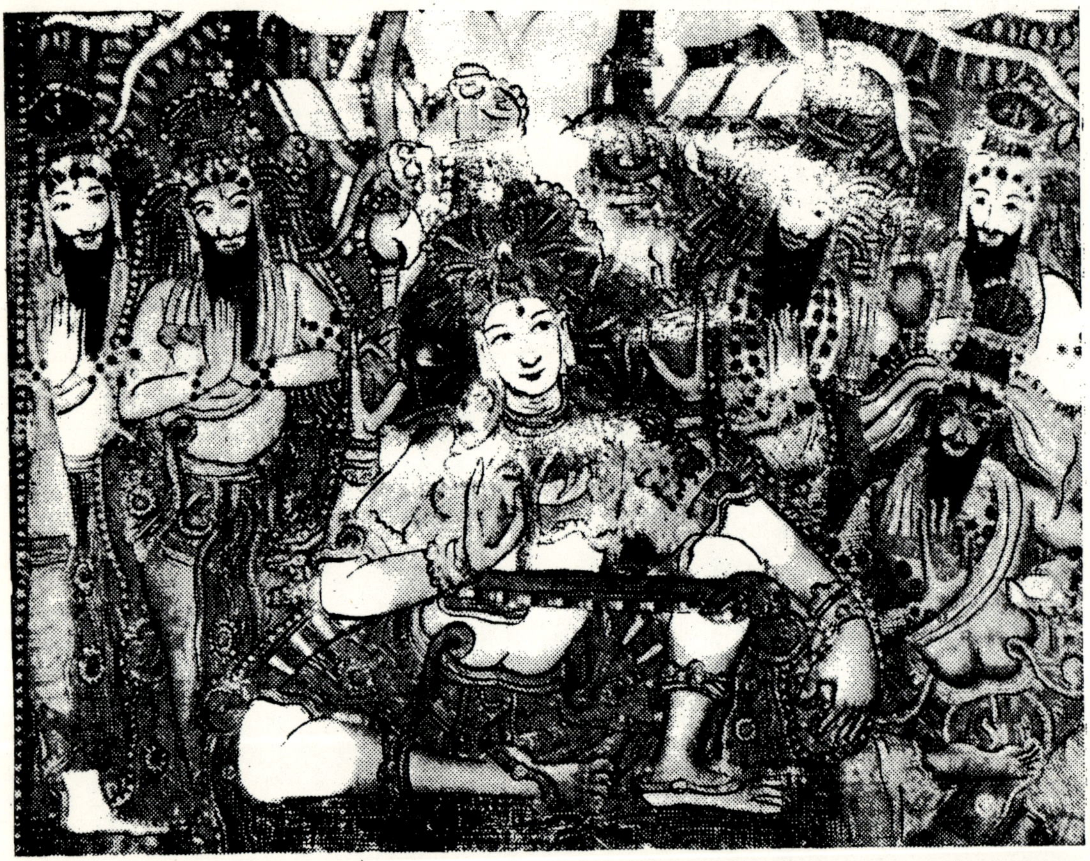

RUDRA as Dakshiṇāmūrti: from a mural in Padmanābhapuram Palace, Trivandrum.

The Historical Perspective

The Historical Perspective

Indian medicine has come down to us in several strands, four of which stand out rather conspicuously. The first strand is composed of professional physicians, called *vaidyas* or *bhiṣhaks* originally belonging to a class of people known as the *aṁbashṭas*. The second consists of wandering pedlars, mostly of tribal origin, who collect herbs and drugs from forests and mountains and sell them in villages. The third group comprises temple priests, especially of the Vaikhānasa persuasion, who are also required to function as physicians. The fourth strand is illustrated by what may be called the 'home remedies', the medical wisdom and practices that were until recently current within the domestic set-up as "grandmother's prescriptions" all over the country.

It is needless to say that all the four strands have unfortunately fallen on evil days, and the traditional skill and wisdom have almost entirely disappeared. To inquire into their background today may merely be an historical exercise. But in the context of the present attempt to revive or revitalize the indigenous medical practices in India, such an inquiry would appear not only relevant but also necessary.

It can readily be seen that the first of these strands relies on an elaborate literary tradition and an empirical discipline. The other three are obviously rooted in folk practices and are to an extent shaped by cultic ideas. They naturally lack a documented or standardized tradition to sustain their prescriptions and practices. But considering the widespread and singularly striking correspondence between these practices in different parts of India, it is reasonable to assume that the folk tradition, although unwritten, has been deep-rooted and broad-based. It is possible that even the medical wisdom and skill of the professional physician in ancient India were ultimately founded on folk tradition. The essential framework was provided by the folk expertise, and the details were worked out in subsequent years by observation, reasoning, experience, and also experimentation.

This is not unnatural, for health was one of the major folk preoccupations. Man's concern with his health is as old as his life on earth. That the body should function efficiently was as much of a necessity in the early stages of man's existence as it is now. In fact, the necessity then was greater than now, for man had to be alert enough to grapple adequately with the challenges from nature that swooped suddenly on him. The terrors of the wild and the vagaries of the weather held out risks for him. The food that he ate might turn into poison, and his bones might crack on a hunting spree. His encounters with nature were many and hazardous. The disabilities that his body might suffer would throw him out of the stern race for survival. Add to this the fear of the unknown and the uncanny that has haunted man from his earliest days till today.

Whatever the social status attached to the calling of a professional healer or pedlar in drugs, that the society needed his services has been evident all through man's career on earth. During the early stages, when man's life was more natural than it came to be later, his health would be governed largely by instinct, and his concern with it would largely be a matter of common sense. The remedial measures for the ailments would be intuitively apprehended, rather than reasoned out and deliberated upon.

One of the early medical authorities,

Charaka, has been credited with two statements that are apparently conflicting. One of them is that as long as man lived a natural life, he was altogether free from ailments. There came, in other words, a time when his life was no longer natural, and then the ailments broke out and have been plaguing him ever since. The other statement ascribed to Charaka is that diseases and mankind have been co-existent all along. There was no period in human history when ailments were altogether absent. His reasoning is as follows : Never was there a period on earth when life was not there, and there never was a condition of life when intelligence did not help life. There have been, therefore, in every stage of life on earth, beings who were not only intelligently aware of the unfavourable conditions of body and life, but also of the procedures that would correct such unfavourable conditions. In other words, ailments as also medicines have always existed. Health has been a continuing concern of man.

Professional medicine in India has four major lines of development, all of which go back in their origin to a very remote past. Two of them, one represented by the physician Charaka and the other by the surgeon Suśruta (both of whom lived in centuries prior to the Christian era), are collectively designated as Āyurveda (or the Science of Life), and are sought to be integrated into the Vedic corpus. They constitute but one tradition, eight-fold in details. The third line of development is the system of therapeutical alchemy known as 'Rasavaidya' (or the Rasāyana school), in which the use of metals and mercury is extensive. This is the meeting place of Indian chemistry and Indian medicine. This system, normally included in the Āyurveda tradition, developed almost independently of the Vedic corpus, and profited by contact with such cultures as the Arabian, the Persian and the Chinese. The fourth line of development is the Siddha (or 'the adept') system, the origin of which is largely obscure, but was obviously outside the Vedic tradition; at present, it is prevalent only in South India, especially Tamil Nadu. There can be little doubt that all these systems were rooted in the Tāntrik culture, and were to a great extent influenced by the Sāṁkhya-Yoga complex.

The fear of death which has ever haunted man has been the most potent motivation for the development and discovery of techniques to prolong life : the goal of all spiritual endeavour as well as all the worldly activities of man is 'deathlessness' *(amṛtam)* or continuity of existence. In fact, religions which believe in life hereafter and in the immortality of soul have sprung from this deep-seated longing. The early attempt was to prolong the physical existence itself, to make the body strong enough to survive the odds, to render the body itself in a sense immortal, and to transform the essence *(rasa)* of the fleeting physical existence into a diamond-like substance *(vajra)*. Alchemy, as is well-known, works within this framework.

If death generates a strong sense of fear, disease is likewise a major source of concern. Death is inescapable, but diseases could be prevented and cured. When the causes of disease were largely unknown, evil spirits or malevolent deities, were regarded as causes and black magic, witchcraft and sorcery gained importance in man's imagination. Not only religions have passed through this stage, but even science has gone through it. Medicine, in particular, was, in its early phases of development intimately involved with these apparently irrational procedures. It was only gradually and recently that medicine was extricated from this involvement.

In Indian medicine, the passage from the irrational to the 'rational' was not only very gradual, but in a sense, never complete. It does not, however, mean that in India medicine remained stagnant and tied up with primitive beliefs. Far from it. It made marvellous progress, especially Āyurveda. Its diagnostic methods, therapeutic procedures, employment of a large number of articles most of which are commonly used in the Hindu kitchen, discovery of the excellent medicinal properties of herbs, plants, trees and spices, and the determination of the dosage and the manner of taking medicines were all very well thought out, tried out, codified and systematised.

And more than all this, Āyurveda developed a neat and consistent philosophy, which again is a marvel considering its antiquity. This philosophy is singularly free from 'the primitive mentality' which sustained magical practices. The old ideas of deathlessness, permanence of bodily existence and immunity from all possible forces of disintegration were in Āyurveda brought down to the idea of sound and effective health. There can possibly be little indeed that is mystical in a medical system. But intuition has its own role to play, and many of the basic ideas of the philosophy of Indian medicine were obtained, not so much by reason or observation as by a different process which may be described as 'irrational'.

The exact process by which the ancient sages arrived at the fundamental concepts like those of *doṣa* and its *vaiśamya* is obscure. Equally uncertain is how they identified the medicinal properties of hundreds of plants, or how they formulated the precise pharmaceutical details. The usual methods of trial and error, drug sample surveys, and observations in controlled conditions are of course to be ruled out. There is a reference to animal behaviour in conditions of sickness having given a clue to human beings (AV, 8,7,23-26). But this was naturally in a limited framework. Likewise, the folk acquaintance with herbs, which is mentioned (CS, Su. Sth. 38,5), should also have been of limited application.

Notwithstanding the accumulation of significant data, refinement in treatment methods, improvement in the methods of drug preparation, the ideological position remained substantially unchanged throughout the ages. While the practice was thoroughly rational, the theory remained 'irrational' (in the sense of being beyond reason but intuitively justified). And the use of magical formulae, precious stones, amulets, talismans, and mystic diagrams for curative ends continued alongside an elaborate pharmacopoeia. It is curious, if also somewhat paradoxical, that magic and medicine could coexist for such a long stretch of time in a country that has been for ages intellectually alert.

The two lines of development of medicine in India represented by Charaka *(C.* second century B.C.) and Suśruta (*C.* sixth century B.C.) are together known as Āyurveda, and go back to an uncertain antiquity. There are legends which seek to establish a continuity between the Āyurvedic tradition and the Vedic tradition, with an assumption that the Vedic tradition is without an identifiable beginning.

Sometimes, Ayurveda is regarded as the fifth Veda (e.g. *Brahma-vaivarta-purāṇa,* 1,16,9-10, and *Kāśyapa-Saṁhitā)*; but it is more usual to regard it as a supplementary Veda *(upaveda)*. According to *Mahābhārata* (2, II, 33 as spelt out by the commentator Nīlakaṇṭha), it is one of the four *upavedas,* others being archery *(dhanur-veda),* musicology *(gāndharva vidyā)* and political science *(artha-śāstra)*. Within the Āyurveda tradition itself, the medical science is regarded as an appendage *(upāṅga)* of the fourth Veda, viz., *Atharva-veda.* There is a belief that this appendage originally comprised 1,000 sections (while the Veda itself consisted of a little more than 6000 verses!); but in consideration of the brevity of human life and the poverty of our wisdom, this immense mass was supposed to have got attenuated in course of time to just eight divisions, the extant *ashṭāṅga-Āyurveda*. Whether it is regarded as an appendage (as Suśruta does), or as a supplementary portion (as Vāgbhaṭa does), or as an independent Veda (as Charaka does), its association with *Atharva-veda* is generally an accepted proposition.

It is well known that *Atharva-veda* is outside the classical Vedic complex which originally was only threefold *(trayī)* — *Ṛk, Yajus* and *Sāman*. Although *Atharva-veda* came to acquire the Vedic status at a somewhat later date, the content is clearly more ancient than the *Ṛks* themselves.[1] It has been shown that the *Atharva* really goes back to the Indus age.[2] Indeed, the outlook of magical spells, amulets, charms, incantations, curative abracadabra, witchcraft and sorcery that we find predominant in this Veda, reflects a primitive mentality which is also to be found in *Ṛgveda*.

Atharvāṅgiras, the old name for the *Atharva-veda* suggests a twofold approach : pacificatory-curative practices *(śānta)* and the practices of witchcraft and sorcery *(ghora)*. Both practices were alike in the hands of priestly magicians and 'medicine-men' (the *atharvans*), who dominated the scene before and during the Ṛgvedic period. The situation has continued till now, after nearly 7,000 years, in the rural parts of India and among the tribal folk.

Kullūka-bhaṭṭa, Manu's commentator, was right when he said that there are in this country two distinct traditions, Tāntrik and Vedic.[3] The latter is generally, but not necessarily, associated with the Aryan achievement of an abstract, other-worldly, sacrificial-symbolic, intellectual-philosophical outlook; and the former is identified with the numerous pre-Aryan folk cults with a ritualistic involvement, especially related to the Mother-goddess and strongly oriented to the satisfaction of natural instincts. There is little doubt that Atharva-veda emerged out of this mass of popular beliefs and practices, in an attempt to accommodate them within the Vedic tradition.

It is highly significant, therefore, that Āyurveda is related to *Atharva-veda*. Of the nine classical recensions *(śākhās)* of this Veda, only two (Paippalāda and Śaunakīya) are available now. The ninth recension, called 'chāraṇavaidya', no longer extant, presumably contained the lore of wandering medical practitioners and also curatives *(bheshajāni)*. Probably, the wandering physicians of this age were responsible for the creation of a school of medical thought, expounded and defended later by the Ātreya-Charaka line of development.

It is interesting in this connection to recall that *Charaka-saṁhitā* argues that there was no time when medical knowledge and practices were not current among the people. Āyurveda, in this view, has a timeless continuity; when it is related or affiliated to Veda it is in the nature of a concession to sophistication. It would be wrong to regard Āyurveda as a development of *Ṛgveda* or of *Yajurveda* as the 'Vedāṅgās' (like Nirukta, Jyotisha, Chandas and Śikshā) were. In fact, it belongs more naturally to the amorphous heterogenous Tāntrik tradition, which in point of time was pre-Vedic.

When we find characteristically Āyurvedic ideas like the circulation of multiple breaths inside the body, or the three pathogenic factors *(tridosha)*, or the medicinal properties of the herbs and plants *(oshadhi)* in the Vedic literature, it is to be assumed that the Vedic culture found it necessary or expedient to assimilate these meaningful or prevalent ideas belonging to the people at large.

It is psychologically significant that Vedic references with regard to physicians and to the medical practice in general betray an ambivalent feeling. It was necessary and practical to accept medical aid in times of need, and that is how medical knowledge was incorporated in the Vedic group, although this knowledge came from the folk that they frequently fought with. Rudra, clearly a divinity belonging to the Tāntrik culture, was the 'first physician' *(prathamo daivyo bhishak)* and the Vedic poet prays : "O Rudra, may we not make you furious! You are indeed a bull! We hear that you are the best among physicians; and, may our children grow up with your remedies!"[4]

Aśvins are again the first physicians who protect and rescue the blind, the weak, the aged and those 'that have fallen into the pit'.[5] But they are impure *(apūtau)* 'like the physicians that wander among men' : and physicians are 'unclean, unworthy of sacrifice'.[6] *Ṛgveda* includes a hymn to the healing herbs ('Oshadhīstuti', 10, 97), ascribed to the 'cure-man' *(bhishaja)* and addressed to Soma, the divine king of plants who is represented on earth by the psychedelic drink (Indian hemp ? asclepiade ?), which the Vedic poets drank and offered to the gods. But the stigma attached to the healing art continued till the period in which the *Dharma-śāstras* were prepared; medicine was considered an ignoble profession which no high-born one should condescend to take up. It was a service which was no doubt vital, but in the vocational hierarchy, it was assigned an inferior status.

Whatever the reason for the initial taboo, in later times when drinking became morally reprehensible and was considered a vice which heralded other vices, the healing art which extolled the virtues of wine (as illustrated in *Charaka* - and *Bhela-saṁhitās* where a good case for liquor is made out) was naturally looked down upon. Ayurveda not only includes alcohol in its pharmacopoeia *(āsavas* and *arishṭas)*, but had use for meat and drugs extracted from animal bodies. Charaka lists as many as 170 medicines of animal origin.

The Ayurvedic notion of a happy life was not exactly to the liking of the austere, ascetic and puritanical law-givers. They naturally frowned upon such advice coming from Ayurvedic sources : "There is no sin in eating meat, in drinking liquor, or in sex-indulgence : they are natural inclinations. But there is great merit in self-restraint."[7] Belonging as it does to the Tāntrik tradition, Ayurveda looked upon body as the home of enjoyments *(bhoga)* and also of ailments *(roga)*. Drinking can be for enjoyment : it is hearty, it makes one light, is good for all beings, it removes worry, pain and fatigue, it expands the mind and corrects the disorders of phlegm;[8] but excessive drinking *(pānātyaya)* can be seriously disturbing. And all Ayurvedic texts contain a section of treatment procedures for alcoholics.

Health for them was of the highest consideration, and proper enjoyment was after all a part of sound health. Clean life, good food, normal pleasures and vigorous health constituted the major part of Ayurvedic ethics : deprivation and over-indulgence were equally wrong in this outlook. If austerity was prescribed, it was in consideration of health, and not because of religious reasons.

And, the physicians naturally attached enormous importance to the body, its preservation and improvement *(yoga-kshema)*. A physician was expected to understand human constitution *(dehatattva)* and human nature *(dehasvabhāva)*; and his job was to secure the efficiency of the physical apparatus that we call the body *(kāyasādhanā)*. These ideas were directly drawn from the Tāntrik tradition. The emphasis on nature and on the need to improve upon it, were basically related to the Sāṁkhya-Yoga complex. The later movements in the Vedic culture which were influenced by the Śramaṇa culture (Buddhism and Jainism), on the other hand, regarded the body as something to be vigilant about, and to be ruled over with an iron will; and they commended the reduction of demands to the barest minimum. Phenomenal existence *(loka-tattva)* was here regarded not only as unimportant, but as a potential evil.

The outlook that gained currency in the wake of this influence, but at a much later period, looked upon the body as essentially an evil, a snare, a home of dirt, a habitation of the satanical forces of lust, greed, envy and wrath; by and large, it was considered impossible for soul to reach salvation until the physical body was eliminated or sufficiently weakened. But Ayurveda held that the body was the foundation of all wisdom and the source of all the supreme objectives *(dharma, artha, kāma,* and *moksha)*; apart from his body there is nothing that is of help to man here or hereafter. If one does not realize the Absolute in this very body, argued Ayurveda, it is even more difficult for him to realize it when he has gone beyond the body.

The antipathy entertained by orthodoxy towards Ayurveda must be considered in this background. And when Ayurveda had to be accommodated within the Vedic complex, *Atharva-veda* was naturally where it belonged. Charaka claims that *Atharva-veda* is superior to other Vedas as it deals with life which is the foundation of all happiness and profit,[10] and this is symptomatic of the sensitivity of the medical practitioners of that period. Their affiliation to *Atharva-veda* was in the nature of a challenge, for that Veda enjoyed a dubious reputation in the orthodox circles.

Charaka's commentator, Chakrapāṇidatta, boldly suggests that *Atharva-veda* itself became Ayurveda by focusing its attention on the curative aspect.[11] The orthodox view, however, was slightly different. Dārila-Bhaṭṭa, an early commentator on *Kauśika-sūtra* belonging to the Śaunakīya recension of *Atharva-veda,* says : "There are two kinds of diseases, one kind caused by eating unwholesome food, and the other caused by evil spirits. The former are treated by Ayurveda, while the latter are dealt with in this science (viz., *Atharva-veda*)."[12]

Diseases caused by unnatural conditions and beyond easy or precise diagnosis were generally ascribed to the wrath of spirits, infection of unwholesome elements, influence of evil forces, effect of magic, or transgression of tribal laws. The treatment of such ailments naturally involved the employment of supernatural agencies to one's own advantage. The curative procedures in *Atharva-veda* includes magical spells *(mantra)*, wearing of amulets or precious stones *(maṇidhāraṇa)*, expiation *(prāyaścitta)*, magical potions *(auṣadha)*, sacrifices *(bali* and *homa)*, pacificatory rites *(maṅgala* and *svastyayana)*, fasting *(upavāsa)*, and pilgrimage *(tīrthayātrā)*. All these have survived in India to this day, despite their rejection in the later Vedic tradition. Most of these practices go back to pre-Vedic tradition, even as the other downright occult practices.

One of the eight branches of classical Ayurveda was the treatment of ailments caused by supernatural agencies *(bhūta-vidyā)*; another was toxicology *(agada-tantra)*, counter-acting poisonous bites and evil influences; still another was virilification *(vājīkaraṇa)*, restoring lost or reduced vitality, by medical and magical means. These three branches belong more naturally to *Atharva-veda* than to classical Ayurveda. The other five branches, general therapeutics *(kāya-chikitsā)*, surgery *(śalya-tantra)*, treatment of diseases of Ear Nose Throat (ENT) *(śālākya-tantra)*, were specialised in Ayurveda : they developed altogether independently of the *Atharva-veda*.

Although Indian medicine sought to wean itself away from Atharvaṇic practices and ideology even at an early age, it retained its Tāntrik complexion for a long time. Even classical Ayurveda accepted Sāṁkhya as its theoretical basis (in both CS and SS), and Sāṁkhya has been shown to be the viewpoint of the Tāntrik tradition,[13] uncompromisingly atheistic and materialistic in its early phases at least, and therefore anti-Vedic.

We find in *Charaka-saṁhitā* in its present

form (*C.* first century B.C.) the earlier Sāṁkhya of Pañchaśikha, whereas in *Suśruta-saṁhitā* as redacted by Nāgārjuna (*C.* third century A.D.) the Sāṁkhya is of the classical type (Iśvarakṛshṇa's). There is, in both *Saṁhitās*, a considerable softening of the anti-Vedic fervour and an attempt to reconcile the Sāṁkhya with the general orthodox orientation. We have to note that both these *saṁhitās* are only reconstructions and redactions of earlier Tantras which have been lost. We can never conjecture what the orientation of these lost Tantras was like. The very expression 'Saṁhitā' in the works ascribed to Charaka and Suśruta betrays an anxiety to fall in line with the orthodox texts belonging to the Vedic literature. Charaka's *Saṁhitā* was a reconstruction of a Tantra, *Agniveśa-tantra* (as in the colophon "ityagniveśakṛte tantre Charaka-pratisaṁskṛte"). Of the 1500 medical tracts listed in Aufrecht's Catalogue, a good many are styled Tantras : *Jīvaka-tantra, Kapila-tantra, Sātyaki-tantra, Karāla-tantra,* and so on. Even the eight branches *(ashṭāṅga)* of classical Ayurveda were called Tantras : *Śalya-tantra, Agada-tantra, Rasāyana-tantra, Śālākya-tantra, Vājīkara-tantra,* etc. It is not accidental that all these were called Tantras. The belongingness of Ayurveda to the Tāntrik tradition has been consistent.

Indian medicine was actively cultivated during several centuries (seven to eight centuries according to Filliozat)[14] before the the birth of Christ. We have the evidence of Megasthenes, the Greek ambassador who visited India in the fourth century B.C., that the Śramaṇas (a group of philosophers and ascetics outside the Vedic fold) were practising medicine and were greatly honoured by the people for this service. There is a suggestion in Strabo (15, 170) that these Śramaṇas *(pramanai)* were also magicians, giving credence to the view that Indian medicine belonged to the Tāntrik tradition.

It is customary to recognise two major lines of development in Ayurveda, one specialising in general therapeutics *(Kāya-chikitsā)* and the other with a bias in favour of surgery *(śalya-tantra).* The two branches have much in common; and the basic theoretical framework is the same in both. The former line of development reached its culmination in the *Saṁhitā* of Charaka while the latter achieved its perfection in the *Saṁhitā* of Suśruta. These two compendia are regarded as supreme authorities in Ayurvedic theory and practice, and their authority has been unrivalled despite the numerous eminent authors who succeeded them.

We do not know for certain if they were historical personages at all. Charaka is said to be a class-name for wandering physicians who were popular even during the time of Pāṇini.[15] Suśruta, which means 'learned', may not in fact be a proper name. However, Indian tradition takes them as real medical authors and they are supposed to have lived during the later Vedic period. The line of development represented by Charaka is called the Atreya school and Suśruta's school is named after Dhanvantari. We are again not sure who Atreya or Dhanvantari really was. It is helpful to follow the traditional lead. Both Charaka and Suśruta agree that Ayurveda was first formulated by the self-born Brahmā, who communicated the system to Prajāpati, and he to the twin-divinities, the Aśvins, who in their turn passed it on to Indra. The Aśvins who are regarded as the 'divine physicians' *(devānām bhishajā)* are described as having cured Indra, the mighty Vedic hero-god when he had fallen ill due to excessive Soma drinking (the ailment later nomenclatured *pānātyaya*). The 'Sautrāmaṇi' ritual puts the Aśvins into close relation with Indra, but otherwise their relation is not very intimate in Vedic literature.

After Indra, however, the lines branch off. On Charaka's side, Indra handed over

Āyurveda to the sage Bhāradvāja, who taught it to Ātreya-Punarvasu and other sages. Ātreya had six disciples : Agniveśa, Bhela, Jatūkarṇa, Parāśara, Hārīta and Kshārapāṇi. Each of them composed their own versions of Ātreya's teaching. The first to compose his version was Agniveśa. It was Agniveśa's work, *Agniveśa-tantra*, that was reconstructed *(pratisaṁskṛta)* by Charaka. On Suśruta's side, Indra taught Āyurveda to Dhanvantari, appearing as the king of Kāśī, named Divodāsa, and he taught the system to a group of students among whom Aupadhenava, Vaitaraṇa, Aurabhra, Pauṣkalāvata, Gopura-raksita and Suśruta are mentioned. After Indra, Bhāradvāja was the founder of Charaka's line and Dhanvantari-Divodāsa of Suśruta's line. It is interesting to note that both Bhāradvāja and Divodāsa have been mentioned in *Ṛgveda* as contemporaries, who were "together protected" (and whose 'routes were made circular') by the Aśvins.[16] This would make Suśruta an earlier authority, for Charaka was removed at least by two generations after Bhāradvāja, Ātreya and Agniveśa.

It is unfortunate that all these early medical treatises have been lost, excepting Bheḷa's, which has survived in a single manuscript, mutilated and fragmentary. Both Bhela and Charaka rely heavily on Ātreya (Ātreya-Punarvasu) and claim to follow him closely. The work of Agniveśa (who was a contemporary and fellow-student of Bhela under Ātreya) is no longer extant in its original form; what we have today is only a reconstruction of it by Charaka by writing the 17 sections of the Sixth Book ('Chikitsā-sthāna') as well as the remaining two books ('Siddhi-sthāna' and 'Kalpa-sthāna'), presumably planned by Charaka.[17] Chakrapāṇi-datta's commentary on this work, known as *Āyurveda-dīpikā* (about A.D. 1050), is very informative. There is another commentary, written about the same time, by Śivadāsa-sena. Our knowledge of Charaka's school of thought is principally based on the Dṛḍhabala's redaction and Chakrapāṇi's commentary.

Likewise, Suśruta's work is no longer available in its original form. What we have is the redaction by Nāgārjuna.[18] He is said to be different from the Siddha-alchemist who lived *C.* third century A.D. and wrote several works, *Rasaratnākara* being the well-known one. Ḍalhaṇa (*C.* tenth century A.D.) wrote a splendid commentary, *Nibandha-saṁgraha* on Nāgārjuna's revision of *Suśruta-saṁhitā*. Ḍalhaṇa mentions many previous commentators like Jaijjaṭa, Gayadāsa, Bhāskara; but their works have been lost.

The fusion of the two lines of development was attempted by Vāgbhaṭa (*C.* seventh century A.D.) who compiled his *Ashṭāṅga-hṛdaya* incorporating the views not only of Charaka and Suśruta, but also of Bhela and Hārīta as well as the Rasāyana system. This work gave Āyurveda its definition. If this medical school has survived as a unitary discipline and as a perfect synthesis of theory and practice, it is due mainly to the work of Vāgbhaṭa.

Another great help in equipping Āyurveda with an excellent diagnostic tool came from Mādhava-kara (eighth century A.D.) who prepared his clinical guide-book *Rugviniścaya* (familiarly known as *Mādhava-nidāna*). During the time Vāgbhaṭa and Mādhava-kara lived, Āyurveda became highly systematised; its pharmacopoeia expanded, and treatment procedures got refined.

The system continued to grow vigorously till about the thirteenth century, since which time there has been a steady stalemate. The beginning of the thirteenth century however "marked the end of an era of growth and standardization"[19] In the medieval ages, the Rasāyana system was, by a curious combination of circumstances, rejuvenated; and the drugs and remedies evolved in this system became incorporated in Āyurveda. Āyurveda as a growing discipline appears to have lost its vitality about this period.

If Āyurveda emerged out of the Tāntrik tradition for an independent career, the alchemical systems of Indian medicine, Rasachikitsā and Siddha, continued their involvement with Tāntrik ideas. It is not easy to identify the origin of alchemical ideas in India. It is supposed that contact with China, the first home of alchemy (around third century B.C.), was responsible for the development of this theory-practice complex here. But the twin objectives of alchemy, namely, transmutation of base metals into noble metals (like gold and silver) and the prolongation of life by an elixir, are suggested even in the Vedic records. Alchemic ideas were prevalent here since possibly pre-Vedic times, although they did not produce a system — as they did in China, Egypt, Arabian countries and Western Europe— until three or four centuries after Christ. The use of metals, minerals, precious stones and herbs for both medicinal and magical ends was known to the poets of *Ṛgveda*, and to the authors of *Atharva-veda.*

Chinese influence was certainly there, especially during the early centuries of the Christian era, and Mahāchīna (the great China or Tibet) was a familiar land to the Tāntriks as well as the alchemists of India. Siddha-Nāgārjuna is supposed to have gone there; and the Tamilian Siddha Bogar is said to have come from that country. Both of them were eminent masters of Indian alchemy, during the fourth and fifth centuries. But it would be wrong to assume that India borrowed alchemy entirely from China. It is possible that cinnabar (mercuric sulphide), on which the Chinese alchemy was based, was first discovered in India : called *darada, yaśada,* or *rasa-sindūra,* it was known to the Tāntriks both in its natural mineral form and in its manufactured form.

Basic to Indian alchemy *(rasa-vāda)* is the Siddha ideology. Siddha is an adept, a Tāntrik practitioner. *Siddhi* is achievement, and generally the expression refers to the eight-fold magical skills much as the ability to become minute like an atom *(aṇimā)*, to become excessively light *(laghimā)*, to obtain everything *(īśitva)*, to subdue and overpower everything *(vaśitva)*, and to suppress the passions *(kāmāvasāyitva)*. There is a classical list of 84 historical Siddhas, accepted by the Hindu, Buddhist, Tibetan and Nātha traditions, which became popular in the twelfth and thirteenth centuries A.D. The first of these Siddhas was Matsyendranātha (Mīnanātha, or Lui-pa of the Tibetans) who is said to have lived in the ninth century, and most of the Siddhāchāryas mentioned in the list belonged to the eleventh century.

But the Siddha tradition itself dates back to a remote past, and was connected with wizards and Śamanas of the Vedic and the pre-Vedic times. The common objective of these Siddhas was the transubstantiation of the body *(kāya-sādhana)*; and various methods were evolved for the realization of this objective. Rasa-vidyā (alchemy) was a method that was thus evolved : it was a physical process designed to make the body an efficient instrument both for material prosperity *(bhoga)* and for spiritual upliftment *(uddhāra)*.

It is said that the element of alchemy was introduced into the Siddha cult by Nāgārjuna, who was himself both a Siddha and an alchemist (and his date is given as 23 A.D. by some authorities while others variously place him in the third, eighth or tenth century A.D.) There is a work ascribed to Nāgārjuna, *Rasaratnākara,* which belongs to the early strata of Mahāyāna-tantras. Another work with the same name (by Nitya-nātha) mentions that Nāgārjuna prepared this work for 'the benefit of the ailing' (vyādhitānām hitārthāya proktam Nāgārjunena yat). This makes clear the general orientation of Indian alchemy within the Siddha culture : there was greater emphasis on the medical aspect rather than on material prosperity. This distinguishes the development of Indian alchemy from that of alchemy elsewhere.

In support of the superiority of this system, it is claimed that while other systems of philosophy describe the state of emancipation *(mukti)* as possible only after death of the physical body, the alchemic system advocates the obtainment of this highest state even while the physical body is functioning. Mukti in this system is a matter of direct experience, as 'a fruit held in one's own hand'. The highest purpose of alchemy, therefore, is not merely to transmute metals but to lead to emancipation by 'binding the body' *(deha-bandha).*[20] There is no doubt that transmutation of metals became a favourite preoccupation of Indian alchemists during the middle ages, and several works came to be written on this subject. In fact, chemistry and iatrochemistry in India developed out of this interest. But work on metals was regarded as in the nature of an experimentation, and the frequent admonition found in alchemical works is : "First, test with the metals; and then, apply to the body."[21]

Mercury is an important idea in Indian alchemy. The word for it, *pārada*, signifies that it helps one to cross the ocean of transmigration.[22] It is also the 'essence' *(rasa)*, the 'essence of Śiva's own body'[23] in particular his 'seminal essence' *(Hara-bīja* or *Śiva-vīrya)*, and therefore the 'great essence' *(mahārasa)*. If mercury thus represents Śiva (the male), sulphur represents his consort Gaurī (the female).[24] The creative conjunction of the male and the female was involved in the *rasa-siddhi.* Mercuric sulphide (cinnabar, *rasa-sindūra)* becomes important in this context.

Alchemists in the middle ages believed that all things in the world, especially metals, are ultimately made up of two principles : mercury (the water element, representing fusibility) and sulphur (the fire element, representing combustibility). These two were described as male and female, and the whole world was looked upon as the result of their union. This is substantially the Śaivite Tāntrik position, and Indian alchemy is heavily oriented in favour of the male-female symbolism; and its peculiarity is that mercury, the male principle, is composed of the five primary elements.[25]

Interesting in Indian alchemy is the preparation of a mercurial icon in the form of a phallus *(rasa-liṅga)*, to represent the male principle of Śiva. There are elaborate instructions in texts like *Rasa-ratna-samuccaya* and *Mātṛkābheda-tantra* for preparing this icon which symbolises a kind of esoteric personality involved in the rite known as 'worship of mercury' *(rasārchanā)*. Usually this icon was prepared with a compound of mercury and sulphur, which was mixed with an extract of Barberia cristata *(jhiṇṭi)*, and stirred vigorously until the proper consistency was obtained; and then it was shaped into a phallic form *(liṅga)*, covered all over with sulphur powder, and heated slightly over a fire of cowdung so that it became hard. *Rasa-ratna-samuccaya*, composed by Vāgbhaṭa, son of Siṁhagupta, gives an alternate procedure for the preparation of *rasa-liṅga* : gold and lead, three *nishkas* in weight, and mercury, nine *nishkas*, are rubbed with acids for three hours and the amalgam is shaped into a *liṅga.*[26] This *liṅga* is installed in the alchemist's laboratory *(rasa-śālā)* and worshipped for both material prosperity and immortality. This worship is said to be more efficacious than worship of *liṅgas* at Banaras and other holy places.[27]

It has been pointed out that the *liṅga*, which is the creative emblem, is associated with mercuric sulphide (cinnabar, *rasa-sindūra*). In fact, the Tamil word, *liṅga* means only this substance. In Chinese alchemy, this is described as a compound of *yang* and *yin* (male and female). It is interesting to note that in the ceremony known as *Ashṭabandha* employed in the installation of icons in temples in India, this substance is one of the eight constituents. This provides an important clue to the origin of *liṅga* worship in India, and the Śaivite-Tāntrik cults, that prevailed before iconic worship became accepted by the Vedic tradition, were no doubt greatly influenced by alchemic ideas, especially the male-female symbolism. The usual form that the *liṅga* takes in the classical period is always in conjunction with the *yonī* (female procreative organ) as the base, and the *liṅga* is a symbol of not only Śiva but Śiva-Śakti, the two being regarded as inseparable. The early *liṅgas*, however, were merely erect pillars or posts in shape *(sthāṇu)* symbolising the upward sperm *(ūrdhva-retas)* and the *rasa-liṅga* of the alchemists probably supplied the prototype.

Curious is the employment of the expression 'karma-yoga' in connection with what is known as the 'fixation of mercury'.[28] This yoga is said to work with mercury on the one hand, and with wind on the other; both are to be 'bound' so as to yield the desired results. The Indian alchemists speak of 'swooning of mercury' *(mūrchhana)* and 'killing of mercury' *(māraṇa)*. The former is to transform mercury into a multicoloured substance, devoid of excessive fluidity and mobility; and the latter is to deprive mercury of wetness, thickness, brightness, heaviness and mobility. Its natural state is removed from it so that it could be ingested into the body without harm or danger. It is usual to list 18 processes *(saṁskāras)* by means of which mercury is transformed into an article of utility and absorption. Mercury, when properly treated, can be assimilated into the human system and can rejuvenate it. Working with the wind means regulating the breath and suspending it *(prāṇāyāma)*, a yogic technique. The twin techniques not only preserve the body but make it a 'glorious one' *(divya-tanu)*. A 'glorious' body is the necessary precondition for 'salvation' here and now, in this very body and in this very life. It is in this sense that alchemy was considered as an adjunct of Yoga : if Yoga worked with troubles inherent to mind, alchemy dealt with the removal of the natural infirmities of the body. It is significant that Patañjali, the earliest authority on Yoga, is also considered an alchemist.[29]

The employment of mercury for its uncanny therapeutic effect on the organic juices *(rasa)* within the body was attempted early. The word *rasa* meant not only the juices of the body which are responsible for blood and other *dhātus*, but also fluid extractions and concentrated decoctions. Rasāyana signifies in Ayurveda 'the way of the fluids or juices', which are effective in preventing aging and in prolonging life. In the early phase of medical thought, the fluids and juices referred to herbal extractions and mineral preparations; but in due course, they meant exclusively mercurial medicines.[30] Ayurveda developed the art of combining metals with herbs in the preparation of medicines; and it was known as *kalā (dhātvaushadhīnām saṁyogakriyā)*.

NOTES AND REFERENCES

1. S.N. Dasgputa, *A History of Indian Philosophy*. Vol.II, Second impression, Cambridge. The Syndics of the Cambridge University Press, 1952, pp.280-81.

2. K.N. Sastri, *New Light on the Indus Civilization,* Vol.II, Delhi, Atma Ram & Sons, 1965, p.67

3. On *Manu,* 2,1. (He calls them Śruti)

4. *Ṛgveda,* 2,33,4

   मा त्वा रुद्र चक्रधामा नमोभिर्मा दुष्टुती वृषभ मा सहूनी ।
   उन्नो विरमपर्य भेषजेर्भिषक्तमं त्वा भिषजं शृणोमि ॥

5. *Ibid,* 10,39,3.

   अमाजुराद्‌भवथो युवं भगोऽनाशोश्विद्‌वितारापमस्य चित् ।
   अन्धस्य चित्रासत्या कृशस्य चिद्युवामिदाहूर्भिषजा रुतस्य चित ॥

6. *Taittirīya — Samhitā,* 6,4,9

   तौ देवा अब्रुवन् अपूतौ वा इमौ मनुष्यचरौ भिषजाविति ।
   तस्माद्‌ब्राह्मणेन भेषजं न कार्यं; अपूतो ह्येषोऽमेध्यो यो भिषक् ॥

7. न मांसभक्षणे दोषो न मद्ये न च मैथुने ।
   प्रवृत्तिरेषा भूतानां निवृत्तिस्तु महाफला ॥

8. *Bhela-samhitā,* Chikitsāsthāna, 30.

9. आयतनं विद्यानां मूलं धर्मार्थकाममोक्षाणां ।
   श्रेयः परं किमन्यत् शरीरमजरामरं विहायैकं ॥
   अस्मिन्नेव शरीरे येषांपरमात्मनो स वेद ।
   देहत्यागादूर्ध्वं तेषां तद्‌ब्रह्म दूरतरम्

10. *Charaka-samhitā,* 1,1,42.

11. अथर्ववेदस्य आयुर्वेदत्वमुक्तं भवति ।
    अथर्ववेदैकदेश एवायुर्वेदः ॥

12. Dārila-Bhaṭṭa on *Kauśika-sūtra, 25,2.*

    द्विप्रकारा व्याधयः अहारनिमित्ता अशुभनिमित्ता चेति ।
    तत्र आहारसमुत्थानां वैषम्य आयुर्वेद चकारः
    अधर्मसमुत्थानां तु शास्त्रमिदमुच्यते ॥

13. Deviprasad Chattopadhyaya, *Lokayata, A study in Ancient Indian Materialism,* New Delhi, People's Publishing House. 1959, p.360.

14. J. Filliozat, *The Classical Doctrine of Indian Medicine,* Delhi, Munshiram Manoharlal. 1964, p.194.

15. For he has a special sutra: कठचरकाल्लुक् (४, ३, १०७)

16. *Rgveda,* 1,116,18,

    याद्यातं दिवोदासाय वर्तिर्भरद्वाजायाश्विना हयन्ता ।
    रवेदुवार सचनो रथो वां वृषभश्च शिशुनां मारश्च युक्ता ॥

17. तत्रेतान् कपिलबलः शेषान् दृढबलोऽकरोत् ।
    तन्त्रस्यास्य महार्थस्य पूरणार्थं यथायथम् ॥

18. उपदिष्टा तु सम्यग् धन्वन्तरिमहर्षिणा ।
    सुश्रुताय सुशिष्याय लोकानां हितवाञ्छया ॥
    सर्वत्र भुवि विख्याता नाम सुश्रुतसंहिता ।
    आयुर्वेदयत्रयीमध्ये श्रेष्ठा मान्या तथोत्तमा ॥
    सा च नागार्जुनेनैव ग्रथिता ग्रन्थरूपतः।

19. D.M. Bose *et al. A Concise History of Science in India,* New Delhi, Indian National Science Academy, 1971, p.262.

20. Cf. Mādhava's Sarvadarśana-saṁgraha, 'Raseśvara-darśana' 8.

    न च रसशास्त्रं धातुवादार्थमेवेति मन्तव्यं, देहबन्धद्वारा
    मुक्तेरवेपरमप्रयोजनत्वात् ॥

    'Dehabandha' is in imitation of 'rasabandha' (fixation of mercury by destroying its fluidity).

    पूर्व लोहे परिक्षेत, पद्देहे प्रयोजयेदित ।
    ...यथा लोहे तथा देहे कर्तव्यः ।

22. Rasārṇava

    पारदो गदितो यस्मात्परार्थसाधकोत्तमैः ।
    रसस्य पारदत्वं संसारपारप्रापणहेतुत्वात् ॥

23. Ibid.

    मम देहरसो यस्माद्रसस्तेनायमुच्यते ।

24 अभ्रकस्तव बीजं तु मम बीजं तु पारदः
   अनयोमेलनं देवि मृत्युदारिद्र्यनाशनम् ॥

25. *Ibid.*

    पञ्चभूतात्मकं सतस्तिष्ठत्येव सदाशिवः ।

26. Rasa-ratna-samucchaya 6, 16.

    निष्कत्रयं हेमपत्रं रसेद्रं नवनिष्ककं ।
    अम्लेन मर्दयेद्यामं तेन लिङ्गं तु कारयेत् ॥

For the other method, c.f. D.M. Bose *et al., op. cit.*

27. काश्यादि सर्वलिङ्गोभ्यो रसलिंगार्चनं शिव ।
    प्राप्यते येन तल्लिङ्गं भोगारोग्यांमृतामरम् ॥

28 *Rasārṇava*

कर्मयोगेन देवेशि प्राप्यते पिण्डधारणम् ।
रसपवनंति कर्मयोगो द्विधा स्मृतः ॥
मूर्छितो हरति व्याधीन् मृतो संजीवयति स्वयम् ।
बद्धः खेचरतां कुर्याद्रसो वायुश्र्च भैरवि ॥
नानावर्णो भवेत्सूतो विहाय घनचापलं ।
लक्षणं हन्यते यस्य मूर्छितं तं वदन्ति हि ॥
आर्दत्वं च घनत्वं तेजो गौरवचापलं ।
यस्यैतानि न दृश्यंते तं विद्यान्मृतसूतकम् ॥

29. Ś vadāsa in his commentary on Chakrapāṇi-datta; he speaks of Patañjali not only as an authority on *lohaśātra* but as a redactor of *Charaka-samhitā*. Chakrapāṇi's *Āyurveda-dīpikā* has this verse:

पातञ्जलमहाभाष्यचरकप्रतिसंस्कृतैः ।
मनोवाक्कायदोषाणां हत्रेऽहिपतये नमः ॥

Laghumañjūṣa of Nageśa-bhaṭṭa quotes a statement of Patañjali from his 'work on Charaka'. Śivarāma's Commentary on *Vāsavadattā* has preserved a verse from Bhoja:

योगेन चित्तस्य पदेन वाचां
मलं शरीरस्य च वैद्यकेन
योऽपाकरोत्तं प्रवरं मुनीनां पतञ्जलिं प्रान्तोऽस्मि ॥

There is also an attempt to identify Patañjali with Charaka.

30. For instance in *Bhāvaprakāša*

रसायनार्थिभिर्लोकैः पारदो रस्यते यतः ।
ततो रस इति प्रोक्तः
स च धातुरपि स्मृतः ॥

Definitive treatises of major authors
Popular Manuals
Physicians' Hand-books
and Materia Medica
(alphabetically arranged)

A

Agniveśa : It was Agniveśa's 'Tantra' as redacted by Charaka that became celebrated as *Charaka-Samhitā.* The usual descriptive title in the colophon of the chapters of *CS,* is "in the Tantra composed by Agniveśa, and redacted by Charaka" (Agniveśa-kṛte tantre Charaka-prati-saṁskṛte).

He was, according to *CS,* the foremost in brilliance among the disciples of ATREYA (-PUNARVASU), and the first to prepare the compendium of the master's teachings ("buddher viśeshas-tatrāsīn no'padeśāntaram muneh, tantrasya kartā prathamam Agniveśas tato' bhavat", I,I). *SS* also counts him first among the authorities in therapeutics (kāyachikitsā), according to ḌALHAṆA (shaṭsu kāyachikitsāsu Agniveśa — Bheḍa — Jatukarṇa-Parāśara-Hārīta-Ksharāpāṇi- proktāsu' *NiS,*6,I).

He was an ancient sage, who has been mentioned in Mahābhārata as BHARADVĀJA'S student and as Droṇa's teacher. Son of Agni, he was also known as Hutāśa (Hutāśa iti Agniveśa-saṁbodhanam, *VyMk*). He learnt medicine from Ātreya and crystallized the Ātreya tradition of general therapeutics.

That there was an *Agniveśa-tantra* which survived as such, even after Charaka redacted it in the shape of *CS,* becomes evident by the citation of some verses from the former which are not found in the latter, by ŚRIKAṆṬHA-DATTA (a student of Vijayarakshita, c. A.D. 1239) author of *Vyākhyā-kusumāvalī* (c. A.D. 1288) a commentary on *Siddhayoga.* It appears to have been independently available during *Chkp*'s days. But it is now lost.

Two other works are ascribed to Agniveśa: (1) *Añjanā-nidāna,* (235 verses) dealing with the diseases of the eye, which is quoted by VAGBHAṬA, TĪSAṬA and RUDRA-BHAṬṬA; and (2) *Nidāna-sthāna,* a work on pathology. But the ascription is not confirmed.

Some formulae for medicated preparations from clarified butter (ghṛta) are ascribed to him : Chāngeri-ghṛta, Vāsādya-ghṛta, Tiktaka-ghṛta, Chāvyadi-ghṛta, Tryushanadya-ghṛta, and Shaṭpala-ghṛta.

Alaṁbāyana: An ancient physician of uncertain date, he was reputed as an authority in toxicology. He is said to have classified poisons into five classes (pañcha-visha). His views are cited in later medical commentaries such as *Vyk* and *NiS.*

Alchemy: Alchemy is a practical inquiry into the *materia prima,* the fundamental substance, which can be pressed into gain, like manipulation and transmutation of base metals into the most sacred and precious among metals, viz., gold. The recovery of the basic material substance as well as its employment for transmutation involves elaborate chemical processes, which are secretive for an alchemist and mysterious for the layman. But there is also a spiritual framework for this secret art, as we find in the early Taoist texts of China, where probably alchemy originated.

The *materia prima* is regarded as dual in its composition: male and female, represented by mercury and sulphur, opposite in effect, but uniting to generate a psychic energy. Exploitation and application of this energy make for the adamantine constitution (vajra-deha). Alchemy was reinterpreted as the technique of transforming base physical body into an invulnerable 'divine' body.

Alchemy was a persistent, if also hazardous, preoccupation among Arabs, Chinese and Indians during the Middle Ages. The word derived from the Arab *al-khimia* ("of the land of Khem or Black Earth", viz., Egypt) signified an Egyptian art. Egyptians are supposed to have practised the art several centuries before Christ; but definite historical evidence suggests that Chinese were the pioneers. The founder of Chinese Alchemy was Tsou-yen (4th century B.C.), although the first reference to the art occurs only in 144. B.C. Arabian alchemy was founded by Jabir-ibn-Hayyan about A.D. 760. European alchemy gained ground only in the 16th century.

It is generally thought that Arabs introduced alchemy into India, but we have numerous earlier references to alchemic ideas and practices before the eighth century. The BOWER MSS (4th century A.D.) mentions mercury; the *Avataṁsaka-sūtra* refers to hāṭaka ('the drug juice'), one measure of which could transmute a thousand measures of bronze into pure gold; *Prajñā-pāramitopadeśa* (translated into Chinese by Kumāra-jīva in A.D. 402-405) prescribes drug and incantation to change bronze and silver into gold. Nāgārjuna's name (early centuries of our era) is associated with alchemy. (*See* NAGARJUNA).

Even Chinese alchemy was acquainted with Indian techniques of 'esoteric' alchemy. Chinese alchemy was concerned with prolongation of life and happiness, in addition to transmutation of metals. The emperor Tai-tsang patronized an Indian alchemist, Nārāyaṇa-svāmi by name, who had been brought to China by Wang Hsuan-tse in A.D. 648; this alchemist has been described as an adept in the art of prolonging life. Another emperor, Kao-tsung, commissioned in A.D. 664-665 a monk (Hsuan-chao) to visit Kashmir and bring the alchemist Lokāditya, who was also skilled in prolonging life. It was probably owing to the contact with Indian alchemists that China made a clear distinction between 'exoteric' and 'esoteric alchemies.

But it cannot be denied that both the Chinese and Arabian influences on Indian alchemy were great around and after the 10th century. Impact of Chinese alchemy must have been earlier, for there are many typically Chinese ideas incorporated into the Yoga and Tantra cults, especially in Bengal, Assam and the Himālayan foothills.

Indian alchemy was essentially esoteric, although the exoteric ideas (transmuting baser metals into gold) were not infrequent in the earlier phase of its development. The word for alchemy in India, rasāyana, suggests that the main technique was the production of rasa to prolong life and restore youth. Although rasa in due course meant gold, and later mercury, the rasāyana that earlier medical writers like Charaka knew, was purely herbal. We have the testimony of al-Beruni, "It (rasāyana) means an art which is restricted to certain operations, drugs, and compound medicines, most of which are taken from plants. Its principles restore the health of those who were ill beyond hope, and give back youth to fading old age..." (*al-Beruni's India,* tr. ed. C. Sachau, I, p. 188). (*See* RASAYANA).

However, rasa also meant gold, which was tantamount to 'immortality' (amṛtam āyur hiraṇyam). In the alchemy of all countries, gold is an imperial and perfect metal, which does not naturally discolour or decay; it is associated with the sun and hence is the equivalent of spirit. In China, gold and jade were plugged to the nine orifices of the dead body to preserve it from putrefaction. But the gold that was prepared by alchemical process was deemed to be more effective than the natural metal. The basic idea was that bronze hidden under the earth would be transformed into gold by the natural passage of time, but the time required for this transmutation would be very long indeed. Alchemy, however, would quicken this process, and endow on the metal certain magical properties.

Rasa thus came to mean the elixir of immortality and also possession of supernatural powers (siddhi), like flying through the air, seeing through opaque bodies, acquiring a body of glory (divya-deha), and transmutation of substances (like stone and metal) into gold. Nāgārjuna, the perfect model of a siddha (alchemist), is said to have produced a mountain of gold during a famine, so that people could buy food-grains from foreign lands.

But the preparation of gold in the early stages involved herbal articles and not mercury. Merutunga (around 1386), for instance, mentions that a lump of copper smeared with the juice of a creeper and heated would become gold (*Prabandha-chintāmaṇi).*

At a later date, rasa came to signify metals, in particular mercury (often regarded as mahā-rasa, rasa-rāja or rasendra), the proper name for which was 'pārada', ("that which secures the beyond"). It was so called because it would enable one to go beyond the woes of life. The expression rasa was applied to it because it could liquefv all metals (rasanāt sarva-dhātūnām) and transform them. Mercury (Hg or Hydrargyrum, the heavy silver-white liquid metal also called quicksilver), as is well known, can absorb other metals forming amalgams. It was commonly obtained by sublimation from cinnabar *(darada, hiṅgula),* its important ore.

Preparation of mercury and transmutation of metals became a favourite preoccupation of ascetics of the Nātha-siddha sect and several tāntric cults, in order to prolong their lives and preserve their bodies in perfect health. A whole school of philosophy (Raseśvara-darśana) developed on the basis of their ideas and practices. The philosophy is included among the major schools of thought in *Sarva-darśana Saṁgraha* (14th century). Liberation from the snares and sorrows of life *(mukti)* was dependent upon spiritual practice, which in its turn depended upon a strong body and long life. Mercurial preparations, which are capable of securing strength as well as longevity, came to be regarded as necessary props of spiritual discipline.

Involved in this philosophy was the idea of spiritualization of the body. *Rasārṇava,* an important source book, recommends restraint of breath (vāyu) as well as application of mercury to make the body adamantine and productive of liberation while one is still alive (jīvan-mukti). Mercury thus became the elixir of immortality and panacea for all ills, the goal which the ascetics pursued diligently.

It is said that the calcination of mercury and the pharmaceutical preparations were learnt by the Indians from the Arabs. But we do know that Indians were experts in several techniques relating to mercury around the tenth century. Marco Polo relates that the Indian ascetics (chugchis), who lived to be 150 or 200 years, drank twice a month a "strange beverage, a potion of sulphur and quicksilver mixt together" *(The Book of Ser Marco Polo,* Sir Henry Yule, p. 365). F. Bernier records that Indians prepared mercury so admirably that just a grain or two of it taken in the morning would restore the body to perfect health.

The aspect of Indian alchemy that survived was the therapeutic one (rasa-chikitsā). It was claimed that whatever disease of man, horse or elephant (nara-kuñjara-vājinām) is incurable (asādhyam, nāsti kiñchit chikitsitam) is easily cured by mercury (rasendra) (*BP,* I, I,). The other aspect (dhātu-vāda), dealing with the transmutation of baser metals into gold, fell into disrepute and disuse. It may be recalled that mercury (a preparation or a compound) was not used in Western medicine until 1699. [*See* THE RASA SCHOOL OF MEDICINE].

Arabian Medicine : The nature of indigenous medicine in Arabia, before the impact of Greek medicine, is obscure. But Arabian medicine that is known to the world, and that contributed considerably to the crystallization of European medicine, was essentially Greek, principally in its Alexandrian version.

Ptolemy's establishment of Alexandria in Egypt as a Greek stronghold around 287 B.C. not only helped the cause of expansion of Greek culture in all its aspects, but served to provide an opportunity for Greek talent outside Greece (which was fast fading in her glory and power). Alexandria attracted the best of the Greek physicians.

It would not be correct to describe medicine in Alexandria as a mere continuation of the Hippocratic medicine of Greece. Alexandrian physicians and surgeons made a positive advance over their Athenian predecessors. Not only were their writings more numerous, they were also more methodical, empirical and rational.

The Alexandrian chapter of Greek medicine was inaugurated by Herophilus of Chalcedon around 300 B.C. He accepted the Hippocratic theory of four humours, the Greek anatomy and pulse examination. But another Greek who was associated with the stabilization of the Alexandrian school, Erasistratus of Chios (around 290 B.C.), who was a physician as well as a surgeon, challenged the Hippocratic theory, and thus paved the way for a new line of development.

The medical school in Alexandria was dominated by the 'empirical' outlook represented by Serapion of Alexandria (220 B.C.). 'Empirical' meaning experiential, from 'empeiria' (experience), the school emphasized the approach to treatment by way of observation of symptoms *(autopsy)*, consultation of the records and the experiences of other physicians *(historia)*, and trials based on one's own experience and the experience of others *(peria)*.

However, the Alexandrian interlude was short-lived. It drew to a close when during the days of the last Ptolemy Physcon (145-116 B.C.) the power of Alexandria weakened. The excellent library of Alexandria was destroyed when the armies of Julius Caesar (48-47 B.C.) attacked the town. The physicians, surgeons, medical writers and translators lost their main academic prop. When Roman ascendency was felt in Egypt, Alexandrian medicine shifted its base to Rome. Medicine, became Graeco-Roman in outlook during the first century A.D.

The second century saw the rise of Claudius Galen (A.D. 131-201), the medical genius. He had studied in Alexandria, and travelled in Greece before he settled down in Rome around A.D. 162. He was physician royal to the Antonine emperor, Marcus Aurelius (A.D. 161-180). He wrote as many as 500 treatises on medical subjects, and became an authority for well over a thousand years. Besides his contributions to experimental physiology and anatomy, his theory of the three-fold *pneuma* (spirit) became celebrated.

The pneuma was constantly renewed in the body from breathing the air through the lungs and sucking it through the skin-pores: this constant renewal made possible the continuance of vital functions. He distinguished between the 'natural' pneuma (located in liver and distributed all over the body through veins), the 'vital' pneuma (located in the left ventricle and distributed through the heart and the arteries) and the 'animal' pneuma (located in the brain, and distributed through the nervous system), which together constituted the foundation for the physiological system.

Despite his contributions to medical theory, his therapeutics was closely modelled after Hippocrates. A combination of Galen's theory and Hippocratic practice became the essential framework of Arabian medicine, when after the collapse of the Roman empire, physicians and surgeons first flocked in Constantinople and then spread to Mesopotamia, Persia and Arabia.

The immediate background for Arabian medicine was in Persia, where the Nestorians (East Syrians) had established the Greek medical theory and practice. Nestoris, the Syrian monk who was the patriarch of Constantinople and had begun translating Greek works into Syriac, fled in A.D. 428 to Persia to escape persecution. The Nestorian school of Edessa inherited and represented the Hippocratic tradition as redacted by Galen. The Nestorians were Greek enthusiasts.

This school ceased to function around A.D. 480 when the political atmosphere became intolerable; and the medical experts moved over to Jundi-Shapur, which was another centre for medical education. Medical writers and translators who contributed to the celebrity of this centre were in course of time attracted to Baghdad, when Abdulla-Abul-Abbas inaugurated the Abbasid Caliphate (also known as the Eastern Caliphate) there in A.D. 750. It was the second Calipha Al-Mansur Abu Jafer, who founded the city of Baghdad and established a medical centre there on the lines of the Jundi-Shapur centre. He was an admirer of Persian culture, and encouraged Christian physicians.

During the rule of the three Caliphas (Al-Mansur, Harun-ul-Rashid and Al 'A-Min) Baghdad became a famous centre for physicians and surgeons. Translations of Greek classics like *Corpus Hippocraticum*, Graeco-Roman manuals like Galen's works, and Sanskrit medical works (like *CS, SS, MN, AS, AHr*) were carefully done into Arabic; and the translators included Syrians, Hebrews and Persians.

Among the translators, Jurjes, Yuhanna (A.D. 777-857, also known as Janus Damascenes) and his student Abu-Sayad-Hunayn (A.D. 809-877 Johannitius) were celebrated for their extensive, meticulous and excellent translations of the classics into both Syriac and Arabic. The last, in fact, has been hailed as the 'Erasmus of the Arabian renaissance'.

The translations paved the way for the rise of that remarkable 'prince among Arabian physicians', Abu-Bakr, Md.-ibn-Zakaria-al-Raze, more famous as Rhazes (865-925), who attempted an integration of Hippocratic practice with the theoretical innovations of Galen. He studied in Baghdad and became renowned by his encyclopaedic work *Al-Hawi (Liber continens),* a compendium of Graeco-Arab medicine principally following Galen but incorporating numerous details from Indian medical texts. He quotes from *SS* often, and his teacher al-Tabbari, quotes both *CS* and *SS* in his *Paradise of wisdom (Firdaus-al Hikamat).* Rhazes was well known for his studies on the effect of mercury on human body, and for his work on small-pox and measles.

A short work of his, *Ber-us-sa-aw (Cure in an Hour)* in 24 short sections, is an interesting book of quick remedies for diseases of the head upto those of the foot; the first section deals with headache, and the last with weariness.

A Persian, Ali-Abbas, wrote *Al-Malik,* a medical treatise meant for the princes, in two parts and 20 chapters. It was a comprehensive work on all aspects of medicine. The first part deals with theoretical matters and the second with practical. The book was regarded as an authority for over a hundred years. It was translated into Latin by Constantinus Africanus in A.D. 1078.

The next great name in Arabian medicine is also the greatest of names : Avicenna (whose full name was Hussein-bin-Abdullah-Hassan-bin-Ali-ibn-Sina, A.D. 980-1038, who by all standards was the greatest medical writer in the medieval world. He wrote as many as 165 works in Persian and Arabic; he was also a poet of no mean merit. His *al-Qanoon (The Canon,* or *The Medical Principles)* in 5 sections marked the final phase of what may be styled Graeco-Arabic medicine. He represented a completely rational approach to medicine, rejecting the value of astrology altogether. His works indicate a fairly intimate acquaintance with Indian medical writings.

The outlook crystallized by Avicenna was further defined by Avenzoar (Abu-Merwan-ibn-Zhor, A.D. 1113-1162) and Averroes (1126-1198) who were among the most prominent medical writers in what is called Moorish Spain. The latter's *Colliget* in 7 sections is a comprehensive treatise of Graeco-Arabic medicine.

Medicine in Arabia made significant contributions in the field of ophthalmology, especially with regard to cataract, and also in chemistry and alchemy. The name of Abu-Musa-Jabir-ibn-Hayyan (722-803), familiarly known as Geber, is prominent as the pioneer alchemist in that part of the world. Several new chemical drugs like sulphuric acid, nitric acid, potassium and myrrh as well as many narcotic drugs like opium, belladonna, hyoseymus and mandagoras were introduced by the Arabian chemists and alchemists who worked in close collaboration with physicians and surgeons.

The impact of this system of medicine was felt in Afghanistan, Central Asia and also in India. It entered India around A.D. 711 and since then it has influenced to some extent the indigenous system of medicine. And it underwent a change in India, leaning considerably on Āyurveda. The *Yunāni* system that is prevalent in India now is a blend of the Graeco-Arabic medicine and Āyurveda. [*See* YUNĀNI SYSTEM].

Aruna-Datta : Author of *Sarvāṅga-Sundara,* a comprehensive commentary on VAGBHATA'S *AHr,* he is also said to have written a gloss on *SS,* which is no longer available.

Son of Mrgāṅka-datta, he is assigned to about A.D. 1220 by Hoernle and Gn.Sen HEMADRI, another commentator on *AHr,* cites him. (*See* SARVAṄGA-SUNDARA).

Ashtāṅga-Hrdaya : One of the most celebrated and most often studied treatises on Indian medicine, and after *CS* and *SS* the most authoritative. Written by VAGBHAṬA, it was in the nature of a summary of his earlier and more elaborate work ASHṬAṄGA-SAṀGRAHA, which is described as *Bṛhad Vāgbhaṭa* ('Elaborate V.') in contradistinction to this work, which is *Laghu-V.* ('concise V').

Unlike *AS,* this work is entirely versified, the verses often reminding one strongly of the verse-portions of *AS.* There is a fair degree of correspondence and style between *AS* and this work, although the former is more faithful to *CS* and *SS.* Both the works of VAGBHATA exclude altogether the philosophical discussions that we find in *CS* and *SS* (Sāṁkhya and Nyāya) as well as matters of spiritual discipline *(yoga).* They are strictly rational treatises, and deal exclusively with the principles and practice of medicine.

The purpose of the treatise appears to be to bring together the relevant medical knowledge contained in *CS* and *SS,* for there was already a cleavage between the two traditions, therapeutic and surgical. There is an explicit injunction (utt, 40,84) that neither *CS* nor *SS* should be studied and relied upon exclusively; the two must judiciously be combined by the practising physician.

While integrating the teachings of *CS* and *SS* in one work, the author has also incorporated the pertinent prescriptions of different medical authorities like BHELA, HARĪTA, NIMI, and KAŚYAPA. The work significantly begins with an aphoristic preface : "What follows is what was said by great sages, Ātreya and others" (iti ha smāhur Ātreyādayo maharshayah, 1,1,2). And tracing the origin of Indian medicine to Brahma, and its subsequent proliferation through Prajāpati-Aśvins-Indra-Atriputra

(Ātreya) and other sages — Agniveśa and others who prepared their own medical texts, the author mentions that medical knowledge became 'exceedingly diffused' *(ati-viprakīrna)*; and he sets out to cull out the most essential aspects of all these diversified teachings *(sāra-tarocchayah kriyate)* in this work, which would be neither too concise nor too prolix *(nāti-saṁkshepa-vistaram,* v.5).

There is an intriguing statement at the end of the work (utt., 40, 88) which suggests that Charaka and Suśruta are studied although they are not 'ancient sages', because their works are 'fine writings' (or helpful treatises), while the writings of 'sages' (like Bhela) are ignored, although people normally love to study the works of sages (ṛshi-praṇīte prītiś chen muktvā Charaka-Suśrutau; Bhelādyāh kiṁ na pathyante tasmād grāhyam subhāshitam). Here is the suggestion that neither Charaka nor Suśruta was considered as an ancient personage during Vāgbhaṭa's days; but both of them appear to have dominated the medical scene, pushing the 'sages' into oblivion. What matters, therefore (according to Vāgbhata), is relevance, and not mere antiquity.

This work follows the general plan of *AS,* and is divided into 6 books *(Sthānas)* and 120 chapters in all : Bk 1 *(Sūtra-Sth.)* 30 chapters, Bk 2 *(Śārīra-Sth.)* 6 chapters, Bk 5 *(Kalpa-siddhi Sth.)* 6 chapters, Bk 6 *(Uttara-Sth.)* 40 chapters. (*See* ASHTANGASAMGRAHA for content analysis).

That the book is merely an abridgement of *AS* is stated by the author himself *(Utt.Sth.,* 40,80) : "The *AS* was prepared from the eight-fold medical lore, as ambrosia was obtained from churning the great ocean. Then, in order to help the students incapable of great effort, this short treatise *(tantra)* was separately prepared on the basis of that elaborate work (viz., *AS, tasmāt*)". Again, the last verse of the work explains that this work is called the "Heart" (hrdayam etat) in the sense of essence or core (hṛdayam iva) of all the Āyurvedic lore (ibid, v.89).

The work probably crystallized for the first time the concept of three doshas in Indian medicine, although the thought-structure is as old as *RV,* and both *CS* and *SS* formulate elaborate theories pertaining to it. This work gives, at the very commencement, a clear and simple framework for the dosha-concept as involved in disease and medicine (*Sū.Sth.,* I,6-12). The relationship between the six tastes (rasa) and dosha in treatment is also mentioned (ibid, v.15-16).

It is probable that the author was connected with some royal court (although not the court of Bhoja in the 11th century as Cordier suggests), for he discusses in great detail the functions of a royal physician who is called 'the custodian of life' (prānā-chārya) and whose duties are meticulously enumerated.

Although a Buddhist in general outlook, VĀGBHAṬA freely recommends meat (including beef) as an article of food (*Sū.Sth.,* Ch. 6) and extols the merits of alcoholic liquors (ibid, 5,62, ff madya-varga).

The work is devoid of references to opium, pulse-examination and metallurgical preparations. Mercury is mentioned in passing. Mineral and natural salts are involved in prescriptions.

In the Tibetan Canon, Tan-gyur (about 8th century), is included a translation of this work, along with those of *CS* and *SS* (Csoma de Kóros). It was also translated into Arabic about the same time under orders from the Baghdad Caliphas. It is translated into German by LUISE HILGENBURG and WILIBALD KIRFEL (BRILL, LEIDEN).

Among the early editions of this work are by ANNA MORESHWAR KUNTE (1880), JIBANANDA VIDYASAGAR (1882), GANESH SAKHARAM SARMA (1889), KAILASH CHANDRA SENGUPTA (1890), G.K. GARDE (1891), and SHANKAR DAJI SHASTRI PADAY

(1900 Nirnaya Sāgar).

This work has as many as 37 commentaries, the largest number for any early medical classic. The earliest extant among them is also the most illumining and most often printed, *Sarvāṅga-Sundarā* (or *Sundarī*) by ARUṆA-DATTA (about A.D. 1200) (ed. by VIJAYA RATNA SEN-GUPTA, Calcutta, 1888 and ANNA MORESHWAR KUNTE, Bombay, 1889). There are references to the commentary of JAIJJAṬA, who is reputed to be VĀGBHAṬA'S own student; but it has not come down to us.

HEMĀDRI'S *Āyurveda-Rasāyana* (between 1271 and 1309) is another celebrated commentary on this work (ed. by HARI-ŚASTRI PARADKAR, Nirṇaya Sāgar, Bombay, 1939). It contains only Sūtra-Sth. and Kalpa-Sth. completely and some portions of Nidāna-Sth. and Chikitsita-Sth.

Other commentaries either still in Mss, or known only in references include CHANDRANANDANA'S *Padārtha-Chandrikā* (Aufrecht; Mss with HARI-ŚASTRI PARADKAR, quoted by ḌALLHAṆA and HEMĀDRI and anterior to 10th century), ĀŚADHARA'S *Uddyota* (about 1240, not available), TOḌARA-MALLA'S *Manojñā* (c.1556-1605), DĀMODARA'S *Saṅketa-mañjarī, Hṛdaya-prabodhikā* (Burnell) and *Pathya*.

There is a compilation of drugs mentioned in this work, giving also synonyms, *Ashṭāṅga-Nighaṇṭu,* of uncertain date. It contains a Telugu gloss. Another compilation of technical terms used in this work is *Ashṭāṅga-hṛdaya-kosha* by Valapad K.M. Vaidya (1936).

Ashṭāṅga-Saṁgraha : A voluminous and comprehensive medical treatise, included in the 'Big Three' of Indian medicine (Vṛddha-trayī, the other two being *CS* and *SS*), prepared by VĀGBHATA, referred to as Vṛddha-Vāgbhaṭa on this account.

The work which proposes to deal with the 8 divisions of medicine (ashṭāṅga) is in 6 books (Sth.) and 150 chapters (adhyāyas) : Bk 1 (Sū.Sth.) 40, Bk 2 (śārīram) 12, Bk 3 (Nidānam) 16, Bk 4 (Chikitsitam) 24, Bk 5 (Kalpa-siddhi) 8, and Bk 6 (Uttara-Sth.) 50. It is the last Bk that justifies the title of the work, for the rest of the work deals mainly with but one division of medicine, viz., therapeutics (kāya-chikitsā) and briefly about surgery (śalya). It is miscellaneous in nature and deals briefly with the other 6 divisions.

The first chapter (named āyushkāmīya, 'longevity and how to attain it') gives the content of the entire work, and specifies the number of books and chapters ('adhyāya-saṁgraha').

Bk 1 (40 chapters) is an excellent introduction to the subject, dealing with health, long life, the source of ailments, food, seasonal requirements, daily conduct, personal hygiene, the nature and classification of drugs, the importance of taste (rasa), the doshās, the therapeutic procedures, surgical operations, and blood-letting by leeches.

Bk 2 (12 chapters) treats of human anatomy, pregnancy, difficult labour, complications, classification of individuals, and prognostic aids.

Bk 3 (16 chapters) is pathology and diagnosis. Several diseases like fever (jvara), haemorrage (rakta-pitta), asthma (śvāsa), phthisis (yakshma), alcoholism (madātyaya), haemorrhoids (arśa), diarrhoea (atisāra), urinary disorders (prameha), abscess (vidradhi), abdominal disorders (udara), anaemia (pāṇḍu), skin diseases (kushṭha), and diseases of the nervous system (vāta-vyādhi) are considered in detail with regard to their pathological conditions.

Bk 4 (24 chapters) elaborates the treatment procedures for the diseases dealt with in the previous Book. Several other variant diseases like tumour (gulma), inflammation (śopha), erysipelas (visarpi) and leucoderma (śvitra) are spelt out, and treatment is prescribed.

Bk 5 (8 chapters), the shortest of the Books, deals mainly with emesis (vamana) and purgation (virechana). Complications of basti are also considered. The last chapter (called dravya-kalpa) describes the suitable drugs and the manner of their collection.

Bk 6 (50 chapters) is the most elaborate one in the work although it occurs as the supplementary section. It constitutes about one third of the entire bulk. The author points out that this portion of the book is meant to 'complete the requirements of the octopartite medicine' (ashṭanga-pūrṇah, v. 66). Diseases of children (paediatrics), treatment of insanity and epilepsy, diseases of eye, ear, nose, mouth and head, toxicology, rejuvenation, aphrodisiacs are treated in this book, thus covering the 6 divisions which are not dealt with in the rest of the work. Minor ailments and management of wounds and ulcers are also considered. New material is to be found here, gathered from different sources, besides *CS* and *SS*.

The work is a compilation (saṁgraha) of information, explanations and prescriptions to be found in *CS* and *SS*. There is little that can be described as original. But the value of the work is undoubtedly great, for it has neatly collected the essential details from the two classics, which are to an extent rambling and discursive. The student would find it helpful.

The work has prose passages interspersed with verses, the latter to be met with also in *AHr* almost in exact correspondance. The work begins with a prayer addressed to the Buddha (Buddhāya tasmai namah). Indebtedness to *CS* and *SS* is obvious and immense, although there is considerable original matter that can supplement *CS* and *SS*.

Tracing the origin and development of Indian medicine in its 8 divisions (Kāya-Bāla-Graha-Ūrdhvāṅga-Śalya-Damshṭra-Jarā-Vṛshaih gatam ashṭāṅgatām), the author describes how the medical works were composed by sages like AGNIVEŚA, HARĪTA, BHEḌA, (BHELA), MĀṆḌAVYA, SUŚRUTA and KARALA representing the major divisions. Each of these, however, was not comprehensive (teshām ekaikam avyāpi) and therefore incapable of curing all diseases (samasta-vyādhi-sādhane, 1,1,15). Should one decide to study all these treatises, a lifetime would pass only in study (purushāyusha-saṁkshayah-bhavaty adhyayanenaiva) ! It is for this reason that the author has prepared this treatise, compiling from all the treatises the essential details, without irrelevant matter, unnecessary elaboration, repetition and other defects (sarva-tantrany atah prayah saṁhrtyashṭhanga-samgrahah; asthana-vistara-kshepa-punaruktādivarjitah, ibid, p. 18).

For the first time in Indian medicine, astrological ideas are sought to be involved in medical practice, however faintly. Diseases which originate during different stellar conjunctions (nakshatre vyādhir utpannah) are said to have different courses, according to the sage Hārīta (ity āha Hārītah), and details of this are cited (Nidāna Sth., 1, vv. 21-32 at the end of "sarva-roga-nidānam"). The idea is neither elaborated nor made much of.

AS claims to follow the general framework provided by *CS*, viz., the three-arms of medicine : causation, symptomatology and treatment (hetu-liṅgaushadha-skandha-traya-mātra-nibandhanah, ibid, 19). His philosophical inquiry stops with the concept of the five 'great elements' (mahā-bhūtas), and does not bother about any other supposition of the Sāṁkhya or Nyāya system. The main frame of reference is treatment of diseases and *AS* does not seek to justify the medical science with philosophical assumptions as *CS* and *SS* do.

This work became popular in South India, especially in Kerala and Karnataka. It was edited by GANESHA TARTE in Bombay in 1888.

There is a commentary on this work by INDU (said to be a student of VĀGBHAṬA) known *Śaśilekhā* (ed. T. RUDRA-PARASAVA, MANGALODAYAM, Trichur, Kerala, 1926). It appears that JAIJJAṬA (another student of VĀGBHAṬA) and several others had written commentaries on this work, but they are no longer extant. [*See* VĀGBHAṬA and ASHṬĀṄGA-HṚDAYA].

Aśva-Chikitsā : A work on the treatment of the diseases of the horses, ascribed to NAKULA; also known as *Śālihotram* (ed. UMESH CHANDRA GUPTA, Bibl. Indi. 1887).

The work consists of 18 chapters dealing with species, anatomical parts of the body, speed, riding, management, diseases and treatment of horses. The last chapter deals with stables; the penultimate chapter is missing in the available Mss. Among the treatments, nasal inhalation (nasya), bolus (piṇḍa), medicated butter (ghṛta or ājya), and decoctions (kashāya) are prescribed. There is a section on the poisons and their treatment. [See NAKULA].

Aśva-Vaidyaka : A work on the treatment of the diseases of horses by JAYADATTA-SŪRI (ed. with commentary by UMESH CHANDRA GUPTA, Bibl. Ind. 1887). It borrows freely from earlier works on the subject by NAKULA and BHOJA.

The Aśvins : Twin sons of Vivasvat and Saraṁyū (*RV*, 10,17,2), the Aśvins were celebrated as 'divine physicians' (divyā bhishajā, *RV*, 8,18,8; *YV*, *Vājasaneyī-saṁhitā* 27,9; *Kāṭhaka-saṁhitā* 27,4; *Maitri-saṁhitā* 4,6,2; *Mahābhārata*, 1,7,15; *CS,Ch.sth.* 1,4,40-47; *SS,Su.sth,*1,14). Their skill in therapeutics and surgery is the theme of more than 50 hymns in *RV* (mostly in Books I and VIII). They were also known as 'Dasras' ('charming' darśanīya; or 'removers of disease,' dasyati kshipati rogān) and Nāsatyas (honest ones, nāsti asatyam yayoh).

In the traditional account of Āyurvedic teachers, they are placed between DAKSHA-PRAJĀPATI, their guru and INDRA, their pupil (*BP*, Pūrva-khaṇḍa, I).

In the Vedic pantheon, they are classed among the 'divinities of the upper regions' counted after INDRA, AGNI and SOMA. Always together, the charming brothers are hailed as the youngest of gods, although the most ancient. Lustrous like gold, they wear garlands of lotus flowers and habitually ride fine steeds (hence 'aśvins', according to AURṆANĀBHA). They also mount an excellent chariot, made in gold by the heavenly Ṛibhus, and drawn sometimes by asses and sometimes by wind, bull or porpoise; the chariot speeds on its three wheels, faster than mind (1,117,2). They also rode at times a 'rickety wooden cart and were laughed at by the wicked Vṛtra' (cf. Skanda-svāmin's legend, 1,119,5).

Their office is to heal the gods, providing them with youth, light and delight, and, on occasions, with new limbs and organs. But they also hurry to the humans who are sick, weak, blind or broken, eager to help them and heal their wounds (8,22,10; 2,39,2). Many are their mercies which are recounted in *RV* (also in *CS, Chi.sth.*1,4,40-47). They are described as compassionate and quick to come to succour.

They restored youth to the sage CHYAVANA who had become old, worn out and ugly (1,116,10; 1,117,13; 1,118,6; 5,74,5; 7,71,5, etc.) They cured the blind (ṚJRĀŚVA, 1112,8, KĀKSHIVAT, 1,116,120, KAṆVA, 1,117,8; 1,118,7; 8,8,20), the lame (PARĀVṚJA, 1,112,8, ŚROṆA, 1,112,8). They relieved ATRI from 'a gloomy abyss' (melancholia, 1,112,7 and 10) and made him youthful (10,147,1). They cured GHOSHA, the daughter of KĀKSHIVAT, of leprosy (1,117,7 and 19; 10,39,3 and 6), and brought the fainted VANDANA back to consciousness "even as a clever wheelwright repairs an old cart" (1,119,6 and 7). They quenched the scorching heat of ATRI with snow, and delivered VĀMADEVA from his mother's womb (1,119,7).

Their surgical skill is also extolled. They

fitted VIŚPALĀ, whose legs were cut in a race or a battle 'like wings', with iron-legs (āyasīm jaṅghām), removed the cataract of KANVA (1,118,7), and corrected an auditory disorder of NṚSHADA-PUTRA (1,117,8). They also resuscitated several people who were victims of accident (like REBHA who had fallen into a well, 1,116,24; 10,39,9 etc.). There are prayers to them from people frightened by robbers (1,120,7). Their compassion and service were not confined to gods and human beings; they even released a sparrow from the mouth of a wolf (1,116,14).

Their skill in dispensing medicines of 'the heaven, the earth and the air' (1,34,6), in preventing old age (2,9,4), in nourishing the body (7,9,11), and in securing health (7,8,19) is praised in several hymns. They are described as especially efficient (karma, skilled in treatment) in removing the debilitating old age (jaraṇyayā nirrtam, 1,119,7). They are associated with an ancient version of the three-dhātu theory (trī-dhātu sarma 1,34,6).

There is an attempt to explain their symbolic nature. YASKA mentions that the Aśvins were looked upon as symbolising 'earth-sky' (dyāvā-pṛithivī), 'day – night' (aho-rātram), 'sun-moon' (sūryā-chandramasau), 'water-light' (jala-prakāśa), but suggests that the historians (aitihāsikas) regard them as meritorious monarchs (*Nirukta*, 12,1,1). It seems probable that they were actual human physicians, who became deified because of their extraordinary skill and unfailing kindness.

The followers of the Aśvins were probably the fore-runners of surgeons of the Dhānvantara School, while the bhishag-āṅgirasas (also figuring prominently in the Vedic corpus) were more physicians than surgeons. Drugs are rarely mentioned in *RV* as administered by the Aśvins, but their 'operations' (1,117,13 chakrathuh śachibhih; the commentator SAYAṆA explains, bhaishajya-lakshaṇaih karmabhih) are highlighted.

The *Bowers Mss* ascribes the Harītakī-kalpa (a preparation from harītakī, *Terminalia Chebula)* to them (Chap. II cf. *HIM,* Vol. I, pp. 161-164). In later manuals, there are about 40 formulae in their name (like medicated ghee from Allium sepa, laśunaka-ghṛta; anti-febrile ghee, jvara-hara-ghṛta; anti-toxic ghee, visha-hara-ghṛta; a citrus pill, mātuluṅga-guḍika; turmeric powder, haridrā-chūrṇa; a tonic with piper longum, pippalī-rasāyana; and so on).

Atharva-Veda : Like *Ṛg Veda* (and unlike *Yajur Veda* and *Sāma Veda*), the *Atharva Veda* represents an independent *Saṁhitā.* But the collection of hymns is both heterogeneous and haphazard. It had originally nine recensions, two of which have survived; *Śaunaka* and *Paippalāda.* The former, which is more commonly current, has 730 hymns (sūktas) in 20 sections (kāṇḍas), with a total of 5987 verses and prose passages. Some of the verses (about 16 per cent) are borrowed from *RV.*

The chief concern of this corpus is the daily life of the people, although philosophical speculations are not absent. Naturally, therefore, health and sickness figure prominently. Besides the hymns that seek to secure long life and health (āyushyāṇi) and happiness and general welfare (paushṭikāni), there are hymns that deal with political matters (rāja-karmāṇi), domestic and social harmony (saumanasyāni), spells concerning women (strī-karmāṇi). However, the major theme seems to be black magic and sorcery (ābhichārikāṇi), exorcism and counter-exorcism (kṛtya-parihārāṇi).

Medicine is involved within this framework. But distinctly medical matters (diseases, drugs, treatments, preparations) are so numerous and important that the corpus was designated as Bhaishajya-Veda (Medical Veda) (- Atharva vedo vedah so'yam iti bheshajam nigadet, *Śāṅkhāyana-śrauta-sūtra,* 16,2,1; Ṛchah sāmāni bheshajā yajūṁshi hotra brūma, *AV*, 11,6,14; bheshajam vā ātharvaṇāni, *Pañcha-viṁśa-brāhmaṇa*, 12,9,10; also 16,10,10), although the expression 'bhaishajya' occurs only in *Kauśika-sūtra-brāhmaṇa,* and not in *AV*.

Atharvan, the seer of all the medical hymns here, is reputed to have been a magician as well as healer (e.g. I,2,3,10,11,23,30, 35; II,4,13,29; IV,4; V,28; VI,17,59,85,90, 92,109-113). The other sage, ANGIRAS, who is associated with this Veda, was also a healer; and CHARAKA mentions him among "the makers of Indian medicine" (āyurvedasya kartārah).

It is in this context that Ayurveda is affiliated to *AV* either as a derived discipline (*CS*, 1,30,20-21; ātmano'tharva-vede bhaktir ādeśyā) or as an auxiliary branch of learning (upāṅga, *SS*,1,1,5), or as a minor Vedic corpus (*upa-veda,* Nīlakaṇṭha on *Mahābhārata,* 2,11,33; *Vishṇu-dharmottara,* 2,22,130; *AHr* 1,8,8).

Several diseases are named and described (e.g., fever, takman, I,25; V,4,22; VII,116; XX,39 dropsy, jalodara, I,10; VI,22,24,96; VII,83; leprosy, kilāsa, I,23,24, cough, kāsa, VI, 105,107, phlegm, śleshman, I,12,13; VI,105,107, Chlorosis, harimā, I,22, VI,24, tuberculosis, jāyānya, VII,76,2, scrofula, apachit, VI,5,57; VII,74,76; head-ache, śīrshakti, I,17; IV,12, polyuria, āsrāva, I,2; II,3; VI,44, heart-disease, hṛdāmaya, I,22, glandular sores, nāḍī-vraṇa, VI,57,109, insanity, unmāda, VI,111,1-4).

Anatomical knowledge as can be gleaned from *AV* (in several scattered passages, but mainly in II, 33 and X, 9,1-8) is by no means fanciful or cursory. Structural parts as well as functions have been more or less accurately identified.

We also find the beginnings of medical practice in *AV* (e.g., washing the sores, V,57,1-3; pricking of the boils and applying salt to them, VII, 78,1-2; probing the urethra, I, 3,8-9, stopping bleeding I, 17,4; use of honey for weak heart and bad eyes, VI, 24,1-2; therapeutic uses of water, I,6,2; III, 7,5; III, 12,9; VIII, 6,3; XI, 6-23, etc.; mountain breeze as a cure, IV,13,3, sunlight as a cure for diseases like chlorosis, III,7,7). Effects of parasites in the body (krimī, in the small intestines, ānvantram, in the head, śīrshaṇyam, in the ribs, pārshṭeya, and in the muscles, avaskaram) were known (II, 31,3-5; II, 32,1-4; V, 23,1-5; VIII, 6,15 etc.), as also the methods of eliminating them (refraining, disentangling, removing, fumigating, cf. "Parasitology in AV," *Indian Culture,* II, 99-113). Difficult labour was handled (I,11,5).

Numerous herbs have been mentioned along with their therapeutic properties (jāṅgiḍā, XIX,34, pippalī VI,109,1-6, apāmārga, IV,17,6-8, lākshā, V,1,5, kushṭha V,4, pṛśṇaparṇī, II,25,3, rohiṇī, 4,12, etc). A distinction appears to have been made between herbal medicine (oshadhī) and magical healing (bhaishajya). However, a physician (bhishak) was supposed to be well versed in both.

Four kinds of treatment were recognised : 'magical healing' (ātharvaṇī, securing health by favourable rites), 'witchcraft, black magic' (āṅgirasī, employment of spells to ward off evil) 'elemental' (daivī, nature cure and herbal cure; use of water, air, plants, etc), and 'human' (mānushī, rituals, prayer, pacification, etc). Diseases were regarded as effects of evil spirits (kaṇvas, atrins, rakshas, piśācha, also amīva, apsaras, palala, etc), and disease itself was looked upon as a demon. Charms were, therefore, used against diseases; in fact, a charm was claimed to be more powerful than a hundred physicians and a thousand drugs (II, 9,3). But a charm was often used along with a drug.

Charms are used against poisons also (agada). Apart from poisonous snakes and scorpions (e.g., V,13,16; VI,12; VII,56), poisonous plants (V,6,8), poisonous termites, and poisonous elements in the sun and earth are also recognised (V,13,1).

There are about 6000 antidotes to poisons mentioned. Mineral poison (IV,6) and vegetable poison (IV,7) are distinguished.

Diseases are said to be produced from the three possible sources : poisons within the body (visha, e.g., IX,8,10); parasites (yātudhāna) that enter into the body by way of water, air and food (V,29,6-7); and disturbance of the physiological factors, vāta (VI,109,3), pitta (XVIII,3,5) and kapha (VI,127,2). Animal behaviour was carefully observed to get clues for medicinal plants and herbs (VIII,7,23-26). Medicinal value of metals (e.g., maṇi, I,29 and VIII,5, jāṅgiḍā II,2) and shells like coral (śaṅkha, IV,10) were discovered.

The *Kauśika-sūtra,* which is in the nature of a supplementary text to *AV*, distinguishes (according to the commentator Keśava) two kinds of diseases : those which are caused by food (āhāra-nimitta) and those which are produced from evil influences from a previous existence (pūrva-janma-pāpa-nimitta 4,25). The former are treated by drugs, while the latter are corrected by magical rites (śānti-karma), which constitute the subject-matter of *AV*.

Nevertheless, the *Kauśika-sūtra* contains additional information about various diseases mentioned in *AV,* and also suggests numerous new drugs and treatment procedures : e.g., use of honey in diseases of śleshman, drinking of oil in diseases of bile and wind, inhaling ghee in tetanus and tremor, application of cowdung mixed with turmeric and some other drugs in white leprosy, sprinkling of boiled lac-water over bleeding wounds, application of leeches for blood-letting, use of salt to break open boils, and of the kushṭha plant in consumption and leprosy, and drinking of ghee mixed with turmeric powder in snake-bite (4, bhaishajyāni).

The use of compounds (e.g., ala-viśola-phāṇṭā, 4,25,19), products of the cow, oils, metals, salts, conch-shell, animal products and other articles of food are recommended, besides herbal medicine.

Ātreya (-Punarvasu) : The Indian therapeutics has been designated as 'Ātreya's tradition' (Ātreya-sampradāya), and it was at one time usual for all physicians to be called ātreyas', as surgeons were called 'dhanvantaris'.

Ātreya means "the scion of the Atri family" or descendent of the sage Atri (son of Vaśiṣṭha, and one of the seven celebrated sages in Indian mythology). Atri is a Vedic sage; the fifth book of *RV* has most of its hymns contributed by Atri and the Ātreyas. He was a favourite of the 'divine' physicians Indra and the Aśvins; he is regarded as the first human being to have learnt the art and science of medicine from the gods. *RV* (I, 139,9) would even make him the link between human beings and gods. HEMACHANDRA, however, says that the name Atri actually symbolises the bodily constituent 'chyle' (sarīrastha-rasa-dhātu).

The Ātreya of the medical tradition is said to be a student of another sage Bhāradvāja, who learnt medicine from Indra, who in turn had got it from the Aśvins (*CS, Sū.Sth.* 1, 19-31). The account in *Bhāva-prakāśa* relates that both Bhāradvāja and Ātreya learnt medicine directly from Indra on different occasions. There is also a mention that Bhāradvāja was a student of Ātreya. CHAKRAPAṆI-DATTA points out that some people wrongly identify Ātreya with Bhāradvāja, and quotes an ancient authority, HARITA, to the effect that Bhāradvāja was the teacher of Ātreya (*CS, Sū.Sth.* 1,30)

The confusion is natural because Ātreya and Bhāradvāja were in fact family names, and the two families were closely connected with each other (cf., PAṆINI, Gaṇa-pāṭha, 15, 61 and 62; *Mahābhārata Bhīshma-parvan,* 376; *Bṛhadāraṇyaka-Upanishad,* 2,6,1-3). *RV* refers to a Vasu-Bhāradvāja (9,80,82). Vasu being the usual epithet of the Ātreyas.

Many Ātreyas are mentioned in the medical tradition. Charaka himself refers to three Ātreyas : PUNARVASU-ĀTREYA, KṚSHṆA-ĀTREYA and BHIKSHU-ĀTREYA. It is uncertain if they were different persons or not. PUNARVASU-ĀTREYA is so called because he was born in the Punarvasu (gemini) constellation (PĀṆINI 4,3,34). KṚSHṆA-ĀTREYA is so called because he belonged to the Kṛshṇa-Yajurveda school. There was an Ātreya who headed the medical school in Takshaśilā, and under whom the famous JIVAKA (physician to the Buddha) studied. There is a medical treatise, *Ātreya-Saṁhitā,* which must be the work of still another Ātreya.

In the accepted medical tradition of Kāyachikitsā, the sequence of medical authorities in India is given thus : BRAHMA-PRAJĀPATI, AŚVINS, INDRA, BHĀRADVĀJA, ĀTREYA (PUNARVAŚU) and his six disciples (AGNIVEŚA, JATŪKARṆA, BHELA, HĀRITA, KHSĀRAPĀṆI and PARĀŚARA). Each of these disciples wrote a medical treatise incorporating the teachings of Ātreya. In course of time, AGNIVEŚA's treatise alone survived, being most comprehensive and pre-eminent. Charaka follows this line, and his *Saṁhitā* is intended to be a redaction of Agniveśa's original work; it is thus that Charaka always mentions the name of Ātreya with the respectful adjective 'bhagavān.'

Every chapter in *CS* opens with the remark : "What follows is what the revered Ātreya said" *(iti ha smāha bhagavān Ātreyah).* In fact, the main structure of this work takes the form of discussion-sessions with Ātreya as the principal spokesman and Agniveśa as the chief interlocutor; there are other medical experts who participate in the discussions.

Ātreya is credited with the prognostic classification of diseases into favourable or curable (sādhya), unfavourable or incurable (asādhya), and unfavourable or incurable but manageable (yāpya). In the background of this classification is an interesting dialogue between Ātreya and Maitreya recorded in *CS,* (*Sū.Sth.* 1,10) :

Maitreya : "Medical treatment does little good, for we see sometimes that a patient does not get cured and dies, although well attended to by expert physicians, commanding all facilities of nursing and medicine, and himself cooperating in the treatment. On the other hand, a patient that has none of these advantages does nevertheless recover and get alright. | Therefore medical treatment does not seem to matter at all !"

Ātreya : "No, it is not proper to say so. It cannot be said that medical treatment is useless in diseases which are amenable to treatment. A patient may indeed be capable of recovering his health without the aid of medicines. Even then, medical treatment is not uncalled for. It is like a man who has fallen down. He may be capable of getting up on his own. But should another man help him, he may get up sooner, more easily and without much distress. Even so, the patient is helped by treatment. But it is true that not all diseases are amenable to medical treatment. A physician would of course waste his efforts in trying to cure an incurable disease. Just as an archer examines and decides about the success of his shooting, even so a clever physician must proceed with regard to a disease."

Ātreya-Saṁhitā : This work, ascribed to Ātreya, is regarded as the oldest medical treatise in India. The printed edition of the work (called *Hārīta Saṁhitā*, ed. by K.C. SenGupta, Calcutta, Śaka 1807) mentions that Hārīta is the author, while Ātreya was the master who provided him with the material. Therefore, the work is sometimes called *Hārīta-saṁhitā.* Hārīta was one of the six disciples of Ātreya-Punarvasu, and *CS* suggests that he, like the other five, composed a medical treatise of his own, incorporating the teachings of Ātreya. But the extant *Saṁhitā* ascribed to Hārīta is clearly a recent work, as it mentions not only Charaka and Suśruta but Vāgbhaṭa also. It says that Atri is pre-eminent in the *kṛta* age, Suśruta in the *dvāpara* age, and Vāgbhaṭa in the *kali* age (p.349). This work, further claims that Ātreya prepared five different medical treatises of varying bulk; but Charaka does not seem to be aware of this.

Here is the analysis of *Ātreya-Saṁhitā* prepared by Goldstücker (Mrs. Manning : *Ancient and Medieval India,* pp. 339-42) :

Chapters 1 to 3 may be considered as a general introduction : Chapter 1 relates the meeting of Ātreya with some of his pupils on the northern face of the Himālaya. Hārīta, one of these pupils, asks the questions on the origin and treatment of disease. Ātreya explains that the Āyurveda, meaning medical science, cannot be fully communicated within the limits of human life, and that his pupils must therefore content themselves with a brief account of the smallest of his own compositions, which is contained within 1,500 ślokas (or verses).

Chapter 2 shows the general division of his work into six books and gives their names. In conclusion, it states the eight constituent parts of the Āyurveda.

Chapter 3 classifies diseases, as 1. curable, 2. incurable; 3. curable by charms; 4. scarcely possible to cure. This chapter also distinguishes the patients to whom physicians must attend, and on what terms, and signifies to what persons they must refuse assistance.

Chapter 4 treats of the physical influence of soil and season on age and temper, and on the influence of the winds.

Chapter 5 enumerates the six tastes as sweet, astringent, bitter, sour, salty and pungent; and the influence of each on the human body.

Chapter 6 deals with the medical qualities of different kinds of water: water of the Ganges which comes from heaven; water from the sea; water from clouds in general, and water from thunder, clouds, snow or ice. It concludes with prescriptions for the use of hot water and cold water in specified diseases.

Chapter 7 discusses the physical and medical properties of milk—distinguishing the milk of kine, goats, ewes, buffaloes, camels and women. It states the cases in which the drinking of milk of either kind is beneficent; and concludes by discoursing on the medical properties of butter-milk. Chapter 8 continues the subject.

Chapter 9 deals with the medical qualities of sugar-cane and of preparations from it.

Chapter 10 is on sour gruel.

Chapter 11 and 12 mention infusions prepared from rice, barley and other grains.

Chapter 13 deals with oils prepared from *til* (sesamum), flax, the castor-oil plant and others.

Chapters 14, 15 and 16 also dwell on the medical properties of rice and various kinds of grain.

Chapter 17 discusses four kinds of herbs, according to their leaves, flowers, fruits and bulbous-roots.

Chapter 18 is on sweet fruits such as mangoes, rose-apples, pomagranates, myrobalans, citrons, grapes and the fruits of *carisoa-corrianders* and of the *mimusops eleugi.*

Chapter 19 deals with four kinds of spirituous liquor, as made from molasses, honey, meal and nogweed.

Chapter 20 describes animals as hoofed or horned, beasts of prey, birds, fishes, snakes living in the water or in arid tracts. Many species are given under each division and the medical properties of their flesh are described.

Chapter 21 gives dietetical rules and prescriptions and discusses the properties of food prepared from various combinations of the materials previously described.

The second main division of Atreya's work called Arishtaka consists of eight chapters.

Chapter 1 treats on the moral causes of diseases. All diseases are said to spring from men's actions. All resemble hell, the curable as well as the incurable. And to some crimes fantastic punishments are assigned; a man who kills a Brahmin will be afflicted with jaundice, and one who kills a king, with consumption.

Chapter 2 is on dreams.

The subject of the six remaining chapters appears to be lucky and unlucky symptoms and forebodings.

The third division of this work is called Chikitsā which means medical treatment. This portion treats of diseases in detail. It appears to display much accurate observation, which can only be glanced at in these pages. Intermittent fevers are distinguished as of four kinds returning at an interval of one day, three days, four days or at some long intervals.

Much is said of diarrhoea, dysentery and allied diseases. Indigestion is described as flatulency, caused apparently by overeating; and accompanied by sleeplessness, pain in the limbs, burning in the throat, etc.

The 8th Chapter is devoted to the sound and unsound condition of the digestive fire (Agni) of the stomach.

The 10th treats of sharp pain, especially in the stomach, provided by excessive fatigue, night-walking, sorrow, cold food etc.

The remaining chapters continue the subject of diseases, touching also on consumption and various kinds of haemorrhage.

The last division treats of antidotes.

Āyurveda : Indian medicine has been called Āyurveda, an expression that is not found in the Vedas, Upanishads or in the early portions of the two great epics, *Rāmāyaṇa* and *Mahābhārata;* nor in the Buddhist works in Pāli. Charaka and Suśruta use this term to signify the entire corpus of the medical wisdom. The first component āyuh in the word signifies "life" (jīvitam) and the other component veda refers to "a branch of learning" (vidyā-sthāna).

Āyurveda would thus mean "the science or art of living." Charaka explains it as the science which instructs us about good living (āyur vedayati iti), while Suśruta finds in Āyurveda not only an inquiry into the conditions of good living (āyur asmin vidyate) but also an art by means of which good life is secured and safeguarded (anena vā āyur vindati). *BP* summarises the two views and describes Āyurveda as both a theoretical structure and a practical discipline.

It is interesting that the expression Veda has been integrated with this art and science. The word Veda has several etymological associations. It means "knowing" (vid jñāne), "examining" (vid vichāraṇe) and "obtaining" (vidlṛ lābhe). The import of the expression is that the knowledge is directed towards a specific benefit. It may be noted that the ancient and eminent authority on Vedic interpretation, Śabara-svāmin, insists that a mere study of the Vedic texts will not produce the expected results; and he gives this as the opinion of the 'venerable ritualists' (tatrabhavanto yājñikāh). Veda, that is to say, is not a mere theoretical framework : it fulfils itself only when the procedures that it lays down are followed. The Vedic character of Āyurveda would thus imply the science of life as well as the art of living.

There is some discussion in the early works about the status accorded to Āyurveda. Āyurveda has been variously regarded as an independent Veda, as a minor Veda (upaveda) and as a supplementary text of the Veda (upāṅga). Vedas were originally regarded as three in number, and were later counted as four : *Ṛg, Yajus, Sāman* and *Atharva. Brahmavaivarta-purāṇa* claims that the Creator, when he saw the four Vedas and considered the essence thereof, produced

Āyurveda as the fifth Veda (1,16,9,10). *Gūḍha-bodha* quotes Kaṇāda and speaks of the five Vedas with Āyurveda as the fourth and Atharva as the fifth.

This is an extreme position. Most of the authorities are content to regard it as a secondary or minor Veda (upaveda) or as a supplementary branch of knowledge (upāṅga). *Mahābhārata* (2,11,33), or at least its commentator NILAKAṆṬHA, counts Āyurveda among the four upavedas (medicine or *Āyurveda,* archery or *dhanurveda,* music and dance or *gandharva-veda* and political economy or *arthaśāstra*). KATYĀYANA (author of *Charaṇa-vyūha*) and the 'Elder' Vāgbhaṭa (author of *AS*) likewise regard Āyurveda as an upaveda of *Ṛg Veda* and *Atharva Veda* respectively.

Suśruta, on the other hand, is more modest in his claim. For him, Āyurveda is only an upāṅga or supplementary text affiliated to *Atharva Veda.*

The discussion becomes relevant because Āyurveda as an independent Veda would lay claim to original and infallible revelation, while as an upaveda this revelatory character is to an extent limited, and as an upāṅga it becomes only a matter of secondary or dependent revelation (to use an expression of Paul Tillich).

We may refer here to an inquiry into the validity of the Veda status of Āyurveda. JAYANTA-BHAṬṬA, the renowned thinker of the Middle Ages, in his *Nyāya-mañjarī* discusses this problem. He points out that the validity of a Vedic text is founded on its being the words of a competent, compassionate and trustworthy authority (āpta), known for his wisdom, integrity and selflessness. Such a one would intuitively apprehend and truthfully communicate the truths to others, not competent to apprehend them directly; he is also motivated by a desire to do good. Jayanta-bhaṭṭa concedes that the truths revealed in Āyurveda do not stand solely on the testimony of the trustworthy authorities; they can also be verified by the experience of others. But, he explains, it is impossible for a single individual or for a group of individuals to test and verify the truths intuitively grasped by the sages; and the issue becomes more complicated when you consider the large number of prescriptions and the larger number of their combinations that have become current. The customary methods of analysis and testing become utterly useless. The original authors of Āyurveda were sages, and therefore endowed with the extraordinary powers of intuition and vision. Their knowledge of human ailments and remedies was perfect; it needs no verification or improvement. Jayanta-bhaṭṭa concludes that we have to rely on their words as we rely on the authority of the Vedic texts, without wanting to subject them to our usual methods of verification and examination.

Āyurveḍa – Mahodadhi : A pharmacological work prepared by the physician SUSHEṆA; hence the alternate title of the work, *Susheṇavaidyaka.* The opening verse, however, gives the title of the work as, *'Anna-pāna-vidhi.'* This is amply justified, for description of articles of food, drinks, bath, anointment, chewing-betel-leaves, fumigation, etc., forms the major theme. The work was probably compiled for the benefit of princes and noblemen.

Dhattūra *(Datura fastuosa)* is mentioned in connection with an aphrodisiac preparation. There is no reference to opium.

Nothing has been known about the author. A Mss of this work is dated A.D. 1682. The work has been cited in *Kaiyadeva-nighaṇṭu* and *Madana-pāla-nighaṇṭu.*

There is a commentary on this work entitled *Arogya-chintāmaṇi* by Dāmodara, son of Vishṇu-bhaṭṭa and resident of Vidarbha.

Āyurveda-Rasāyana : This is an incomplete commentary on *AHr.* by Hemādri (ed. by Hari-Śāstrī Parāḍkar, Nirṇaya-Sagar,

sanity are dealt with. Five añjanas (eye-ointments) are mentioned: pushpa-, rasa-, chūrṇa-, guṭika-, and sauvīra-añjana. Insanity is sought to be cured by āma-māṁsa (?). In this connection, the narrative is as follows (pp. ix-x):

"Saikata, the mendicant in Śrāvasti, became insane. His mind got unhinged. The householder that saw him thus complained: 'These mendicants who have left home at the behest of the Śākya Muni (Buddha) are indeed orphans. Had this unfortunate man been at home, his father would have taken care of him and would have got him treated'.

"The talk reached the ears of the Buddha who at once arranged for a physician to visit Saikata. The physician prescribed 'āma-māṁsa' (meat) for the patient. The patient refused to eat meat. When this was communicated to Buddha, he suggested that the patient's eyes should be blind-folded, and that the prescribed meat given to him. They did likewise, but removed the bandage that covered the patient's eyes too soon. The patient saw the remains of what he had eaten, and at once vomited all that he had eaten.

"When the Buddha came to know of this, he recommended that the bandage should not be removed until the traces of what the patient had eaten were removed from his sight. In case the bandage had to be removed quick, the patient's attention should be focused on a vessel of clean water that should be placed before him; this would prevent nausea. The instructions were carried out and Saikata was cured."

There is the anecdote of another monk Svāti who fainted, being bitten by a snake. The physician prescribed, among other drugs, urine of newly born calves, ash of five kinds of wood, and mud. When the cure was not effected, the Buddha taught Māyūri-vidyā to the disciples, who by repeating the magic formula in the presence of Svāti revived him. The preserved portion closes with this charm, which had been discovered by the bodhisattva in his incarnation as a peacock.

It may be noticed that Māyūrī-Vidyā figures prominently also in the *Bower MSS.* (*Nāvanītakam*, sections 6 and 7). It was a Buddhist charm of folk origin against snake-bite, based on the belief that the peacock (mayurī) is an enemy of the reptiles.

Bhānumatī : This is an incomplete commentary by CHAKRAPAṆI-DATTA (C. 1060) on *SS*, named after his elder brother, Bhānudatta, who also was an author. It extensively quotes BHAṬṬARA-HARICHANDRA, a commentator on *CS.*, and criticises the views of DALHAṆA, without however naming him.

The MSS is now in the British Museum, London.

It is also called *Tātparya-ṭīkā*.

Bhāradvāja : He was an ancient medical authority, who was selected by the sages to learn medicine from Indra (*CS.Sū.Sth.* 1,1, and *BP*). He is said to have gained longevity along with happiness — health — (āyur amitam labhe Bhāradvājah sukhānvitah), from this science, Veda, which was learnt from him by other sages who were intent on the welfare of mankind (prajā-hitam), and desirous of long life (dīrgham-āyuh) and improved health (vardhanam āyushah).

He was the son of Bṛhaspati and Mamatā; and the well-known Droṇa (teacher in archery and sage, in *Mahābhārata*) was his son. *RV* often mentions Bhāradvāja, which perhaps was a tribal name. Among the sages who learnt medicine from him was ATREYA (-PUNARVASU), who passed on the Indian therapeutics through AGNIVEŚA to CHARAKA. *Chkp.* was aware of a view that Bhāradvāja and Ātreya were names of the same person, but he thought differently (on *CS, Sū.Sth.* 1,30); he points out that Ātreya has nowhere been referred to as Bhāradvāja in *CS* (kvachid api tantra-pradeśe akīrtanāt).

BP mentions that he wrote a medical work (tantra) explaining the *materia medica* and therapeutics (guṇān dravyāṇi karmāṇi, 1,1). But there is no reference, anywhere else, for such a work; nor is the work extant. A work known as *Bhāradvājīyam* (Madras *GOML*, No. 13178), dealing briefly with urinary disorders (meha-śukla-āma-lakshaṇaprakaraṇe) is a spurious ascription to him. Likewise a Dravya-Viśeshaka-Bheshaja-kalpa (same, No. 13179-81) claims to contain his teachings. (ity āha bhagavān Bhāradvājah).

VṚNDA and ŚARNGADHARA have preserved a formula (phala-ghṛta) of his.

Bhāva-Miśra : He was a medical authority of the 16th century and author of *Bhāva-Prakāśa,* which is acclaimed as one of the three "minor medical treatises" (laghu-trayī).

Son of LAṬAKA-MIŚRA of Banaras (of Kānyakubja, according to GANANATH SEN), he also wrote a glossary of medicinal herbs *(Guṇa-ratna-mālā),* indicating their properties and other details. This work includes 150 more drugs than what the standard *Dhanvantari-Nighantu* contains. The MSS of this work is stated by JOLLY to be in the India Office Library, London. [*See* BHĀVA-PRAKĀŚA].

Bhāva-Prakāśa : This is a standard medical text-book written by BHAVA-MIŚRA, the oldest MSS (Tübingen) which is dated A.D. 1558. It is an elaborate treatise in 3 books *(Khaṇḍas)* dealing with all matters pertaining to medicine, on the triple basis of 'cause, symptom and cure' (hetu-liṅga-aushadha). It became very popular and was extensively used by physicians. It was not only comprehensive but also of great practical value.

Book I (pūrva-khaṇḍa) is in two parts (bhāga) and six sections (prakaraṇa). The first part, which is extensive, treats of the origin of medicine, creation and evolution, embryology, paediatrics, anatomy and physiology (following *CS* and *SS*), dietetics and pharmacology. It also deals with the practice of healthy habits during the day and in different seasons. A glossary of drugs is included here. The second part describes the medical terminology and measures, the five treatment procedures (pañcha-karma), cleansing and other methods relating to metals.

Book II (madhya-khaṇḍa) is in four parts, dealing with cures of specific diseases. An excellent account of pathology and therapeutics is to be found here.

Book III (uttara-khaṇḍa) is exceedingly short, consisting of but 11 pages in the MSS. It deals with elixirs and restoration of youth.

Largely it repeats earlier accounts and formulae, but the lists of diseases and cures have been updated. For instance, there is mention of 'phiraṅga' (a Sanskrit term referring to a foreigner) or syphilis, which spread in India owing to venereal contact with the Portuguese adventurers. It is described as prevalent in the country known as 'phiraṅga' (phiranga-saṁjñake deśe bāhulyena), and as an adventitious ailment (āgantuka) due to physical contact with the persons of that country (phiraṅgino ṅga saṁsargāt). The ailment is described in its three stages : external (bāhya), internal (ābhyantara) and both (bahirantara). When it reaches the internal stage, it is regarded as difficult to cure. Chopa-chīnī (Smilax china), a drug imported into India around A.D. 1535, is prescribed as a cure. Mercury in the form of Calomel is referred to.

Likewise Soma-roga, a disease of women, not mentioned by Mādhava, has been described with its psychosomatic involvements (śokāc chāpi śramād api).

Another new disease described is "possession by the goddess Śītalā" (devyā Śītala-yākrānta), viz., small pox (masūrī). He includes an incantation to this goddess among the remedies.

Among curative substances, opium

(ahiphena) and almost all the minerals currently used are mentioned. Several new formulae are given.

The role of the Aśvini brothers in the history of Indian medicine has been highlighted in this work. We find here for the first time a mythical involvement of the divine dragon Śesha with Charaka. The account given here is : "During the Fish-incarnation of Hari, the Vedic lore was recovered, and was given to Śesha, who became proficient in medicine that was included in *Atharva-Veda.* Once when he came down to the earth to learn how human beings fared, he found them stricken with all sorts of ailments. Then, prompted by compassion, he appeared as the son of the sage Viśuddha and wandered about the world as an unknown emissary, dispensing medicine and effecting cures. Thus he came to be called Charaka, 'a wandering physician' (yataś chara ivāyāto na jñātah kenachid yatah; *tasmāc Charaka-nāmasau vikhyātah kshiti-maṇḍale,* I,I).

Probably this account preserves an old tradition concerning 'travelling healers.' (For details *see* CHARAKA).

The author himself prepared a *materia medica* (nighaṇṭu) as a supplement to this work.

There is a commentary on this work by Jayadeva, son of Jayakṛshṇa of Kāshmīr. It is said that the commentary was commissioned by the then King of Kāshmīr.

Bhāva-prakāśa-nighanṭu : The pharmacological supplement to BHAVA-MIŚRA's celebrated work *Bhāva-prakāśa,* which has been counted among the 'minor three classics' of Indian medicine (the other two being *Chakradattam* or *Mādhava-nidāna* and *Śārṅgadhara-samhitā*). While the main text *Bhāva-prakāśa* follows *Śārṅgadhara-saṁhitā,* the 'nighaṇṭu'—portion follows *Madana-vinoda.* The work has had an abiding celebrity since its compilation some time after the 15th century and before the 17th century.

The work consists of 23 sections dealing with drugs like harītakī (Terminalia Chebula), camphor, guḍūchī (Tinospora Cordifolia), flowers, trees like vaṭa, fruits like mango, metals (including zinc), cereals, vegetables, meat, food-preparations, drinks, milk, curds, butter milk, butter, ghee, urine, oils, honey, sugar-cane, and terms with multiple meanings (anekārtha-nāma). The work mentions the use of Chopa-chīnī (dvipāntara-vachā) to cure syphilis *(phiraṅga-roga).* The basic ideals of pharmacology have been summarized in a single verse (1,6,196). Plants have been classified (15,122) and the medicinal uses of parts thereof are described with examples (1,6,101-102). The soil is classified into four types according to caste-identifications (brāhmaṇa, kshatriya, vaiśya and śūdra, 1,5,115). It would appear that the classical drugs of Indian medicine were already becoming difficult to obtain, for the work contains an elaborate list of substitute drugs *(pratinidhi-dravyas).*

The work has been frequently printed; and there are also some glosses on this. The recent gloss by Kṛshna Chandra Chunekar of Banaras (1969) is useful.

Bheḷa : Also spelt Bheḍa, he was one of the six celebrated disciples of Atreya, who prepared their own medical treatises (tantra) incorporating the master's teachings. He was thus a contemporary of Agniveśa, whose treatise was later redacted by Charaka. His date is uncertain, but he is assigned to *C.* 600 B.C.

He is cited by the eminent medical writers of later times, such as Vāgbhaṭa, Ḍalhaṇa, Chakrapāṇi-datta, Śivadāsa-Sena, Vijaya-rakshita and Śrīkaṇtha-datta. Vāgbhaṭa calls him a "Sage", *ṛshi* (*AHr* 6, 15), and appears to rely on his work to a great extent.

He refers to Ātreya as his own master (ity āha bhagavān Ātreyah), and gives the other names that his master bore : Punarvasu and Chāndrabhāga. There is a mention in his *Saṁhitā* that the royal sage Nagnajit learnt toxicology from Ātreya (Vishayogeshu vijñānam provācha).

Gandhāra, the north-western frontier region of India, is frequently mentioned in his work. It is likely that he belonged to this area.

There is another medical author Bhāluki, who also wrote a tantra, and who is also cited as a medical authority. It is sometimes supposed that Bheḷa and Bhāluki were identical persons. But NS mentions Bheḷa and Bhāluki in the same sentence among the names of other medical writers (idānīm Bheda-Bhāluki-Pushkala-Vānādīnāmalpa-tantra-vidām...). The two, therefore, were different authors.

Bheḷa-Saṁhitā : An early medical treatise belonging to the Ātreya-tradition, probably contemporaneous with *CS,* if not earlier, it has come down to us in a single mutilated MSS from Tanjore (Burnell's *Tanjore Cat. of Skt. MSS,* No. 10773). Transcribed from an earlier *olai* MSS, no longer extant, this MSS is dated A.D. 1650. Based on the copy, Hoernle got made in Telugu characters, the work was published by the Calcutta University (*Journ. Dept. of Letters,* vol. IV) in 1921.

The MSS, much damaged, abounds in lacunae. It is "a meagre collection of fragments" (Gaṇanāth Sen). There are now only 27 chapters out of the original 30 in Sūtra Sthāna, 7 out of 8 in Nidāna-Sthāna, 5 out of 8 in Vimāna-Sthāna, 8 out of 9 in Kalpa-Sthāna, and 7 out of 9 in Siddhi-Sthāna. All the chapters in Indriya-Sthāna (12) and Chikitsā-Sthāna (30) are available. It is impossible to reconstruct the original text, or to interpret the medical views of the author. The work appears to have the same divisions as *CS,* namely, Nidāna, Vimāna, Śārīra, Indriya, Chikitsā and Kalpa-sthānas. It is possible that contents also were much the same. But there is a quotation from *SS* in this work.

Bheḷa and the formulae taken from his work are cited in the *Bower MSS* (Nāvanītaka) : Bheḷa-yavāgu, a gruel prepared from the roots of five drugs, mixed with clarified butter and oil, and acidulated with pomegranates (sa-pañcha-mūla ghṛta-taila-miśra sa-dāḍima) for disordered vāta; the gruel made by old cereals (purāṇa-dhānya) would eliminate ailments due to disordered śleshman; the gruel prepared from white lotus, blue lotus and sugar (sa-padma-nīlotpala-śarkarā) would remove disordered pitta.

The content analysis of the work can hardly be made. But the gleanings show that the author was acquainted with the 'fourfold medicine' (Bheshajam chatushpādam, 4th Chap. of ? Sth.) : physician, patient, drug, and nurse. There is a prescription against suppressing the natural urges of evacuation, wind, metabolic heat, phlegm and semen (na vegān dhārayed dhīmān prāptān mūtra-purīshayoḥ; na vātasya na pittasya na śukrasya kaphạsya cha.).

A view found in this work is rather unique : that mind is lodged in the brain (chittam hṛdaya-saṁśritaṁ). That the expression *hṛdaya* ("heart") actually means 'brain' is borne out by the description of *hṛdaya* found in the work itself. In cases of insanity (unmāda), the mind as the faculty of sensations (manas) is first affected, then the intellect (chitta), and finally the faculty of determination (buddhi).

The number of bones in the human body is said to be 363, a number that is also given in *Kāśyapa-samhitā.* Some medicinal preparations (yogas) from this book are found to be included in the *Bower MSS* (Nāvanītakam).

There are no commentaries available on this work, nor is there any mention of one ever written. The work had lost its popularity even in the days of Vāgbhaṭa, for he expressly states that medical treatises of 'ancient sages' like Bheḷa were no longer read (Bhelādyāh kiṁ na paṭhyante ......' *AHr.*, 6,49), while later redactions of Charaka and Suśrutạ were popular (muktvā Charaka-Suśrutau *ibid*).

Bhoja : Bhoja is a frequently quoted medical authority and author of a medical treatise called *Rāja-mārtaṇḍa.* The author styles himself a ḳing, and is sometimes identified with the polymath Bhoja, the monarch of Dhārā, aḷthough the identification iṣ uncertain.

The work is in the nature of a collection of recipes and formulae (yogānām saṁgraho'yam), some of which are quoted by Ḍalhaṇa, Vijaya-Rakshita, Śrīkaṇṭha-Datta and Chakrapāṇi-Datta.

Bower Mss : Discovered (actually bought from a pair of ignorant Turkish pedlars) by Maj.Gen. H. Bower in 1890 in a Buddhist Stūpa along an old trade route to China, these Sanskrit manuscripts are an important link in the history of Indian medicine (ed. by A.F.R. Hoernle *Archaeological Survey of India, NIS,* Calcutta, vol. 22, 1893-1912). Of the different texts that are included in this collection, three pertain to medicine.

Written on 51 birch-bark leaves, cut in the manner of South Indian palm-leaves, in Gupta characters belonging to the 4th Century A.D. and possibly by four scribes (according to Hoernle), the MSS are, palaeographically, assigned to a period between A.D. 350 and 475. They are Buddhist in general nature, and were probably carried there by the Buddhist monks who travelled exṭensively in Central Asia during the early centuries after Christ, and were responsible for the spread of Indian culture in that area, which was included in the dominion of Samudra-Gupta.

The language of these texts is old Sanskrit, freely mixed with Prākṛt, reminding us of the language of Buddhist texts like *Saddharma-puṇḍarīka.* The verses are mostly in the usual *anushṭup, trishṭubh* and *āryā* meters. Sometimes the poetic quality borders on the elegant, especially in the section on the medicinal value of garlic (laśuna). There are also charms and spells, panegyric verses and prescriptions.

The medical texts are mainly two : (1) *Laśuna-kalpa,* an incomplete treatise on the value, uses and preparations of garlic (laśuna or rosona, Allium Sativum); and (2) *Nāvanītakaṃ,* the quintessence of medical formulae. The third text, consisting of 72 verses, gives 14 formulae. The dominant feature of all these works are selected formulae for general health and for treating specific ailments.

These formulae are taken directly from three principal sources : Charaka (29), Bheḷa (15) and Suśruta (6); the remaining 44 are from various medical authorities, some named and others not. Besides the three eminent masters mentioned above, the MSS refer to the formulae ascribed to the sages, Ātreya, Ksharapāṇi, Jatūkarṇa, Hārīta, Kāśyapa, Jīvaka, Agastya, Kaṅkāyana, Nimi, Uśanas, and Dhanvantari. There are many formulae in the name of Kāśyapa. It is interesting that the extracts from *CS* in this collection are drawn only from the portions that were available to Dṛḍhabala, and not from the portions that he redacted or supplied.

The most important text in the MSS is known as Nāvanītaka, (lit. 'the Butter that is taken out, after churning the curds') in sixteen chapters. The name signifies that the available books on Āyurveda had been examined carefully to identify and isolate the most essential and well-known formulae of sages (ṛshis), which are collected here. The prescriptions and preparations that are listed here are actually taken from several earlier kalpas and tantras.

There are accounts of clarified butters and medicated oils of different kinds, formulae, enemas, tonics, gruels, aphrodisiacs, collyriums, and hair washes (chap. 1 to 10). Methods of using *Chebulic Myrobalan,* bitumen, plumbago-root are also given (11-13). Treatment of children is the theme of chapter 14; treatment of diseases of barren women and those with children (15 and 16) is also given.

The outstanding matter to be found in the MSS is the detailed account of the medicinal value of garlic (Allium Sativum). There is to be found here praises of this drug which became popular in India probably owing to the contact with foreigners like Śakas and Kushāṇas during the Gupta age (hence the name *mleccha-kanda*). The word, Laśuna (or Rasona), which also may be of non-Sanskrit origin, is derived here as signifying that all the tastes *(rasa)* excluding salt *(lavaṇa)* are present in it (lavaṇa-śūnya or lavaṇa-nyūna; rasona-rasa-nyūna; cf. BP, pañchabhiś cha rasair yukto rasenāmlena varjitah; tasmād rasona ity ukto ...). The first of these MSS, which closes abruptly with the 5th section, deals solely with garlic.

Garlic is said to be an effective remedy for several ailments, principally tuberculosis (rāja-yakshma) and enlarged cervical glands (gaṇḍa-mālā); it increases vitality (rasāyana). Its intense odour (ugra-gandha) destroys parasites (germs, krimi). It would appear that there was then a custom of tying a string of garlic bulbs above the main entrance of the house to ward off ill-health. (harmyagreshv atha toraṇeshu valabhīdvāreshu chāvishkṛtāh; kandādyā laśunasrajo virached bhūmau tathaivārcchanam). The beneficient seasons for the use of garlic are also mentioned : winter and spring ('ayam iha laśunotsavah prayojyo himakāle cha madhau cha mādhave cha).

The MSS contain charms, spells and hymns pertaining to Mahā-māyūrī, Mātaṅgī, Vighna-rājñī and Aparājitā, all Buddhist folk goddesses. The *tāntric* element is discernible in these passages, and it reflects the religio-medical approach that was prevalent in the centuries immediately after Christ, an approach that is not altogether absent in *CS, SS* and *Kāśyapa-saṁhitā.*

We find that the essential framework of Indian medicine (the concept of *tri-dosha,* the importance of digestion in health, the nomenclature of diseases, the variety of medicinal preparations, etc.) can be seen even in these MSS. Among diseases, smallpox, and among medicinal substances, quick-silver and opium, have not been mentioned.

Brahmā : The mythical originator of Āyurveda, he was associated with *Atharva-Veda.* He is said to have taught medicine to his son Daksha-prajāpati, who in turn taught it to the Aśvins. The *Bower MSS* mention that the Aśvins were taught by Brahmā himself regarding the properties of Chebulic Myrobalan (Hoernle, XI p. 164).

He is said to have introduced into Indian medicine the employment of horn (śṛṅga), leech and sharp instrument (Vraṇa-Chikitsā, Government Oriental Manuscripts Library, Madras, 23,132-42).

Bṛhadyoga-Taraṅgiṇī : This is a gigantic compendium in 148 chapters, dealing with all topics concerning Indian medicine. The author was Trimalla-bhaṭṭa, a Telugu Brahmin from Tripurāntaka town (?). The date of the work is uncertain. But he gives extracts from the works of Śārṅgadhara, but does not refer to Bhāvaprakāśa. It may, therefore, be assumed to have been compiled some time between the dates of Śārṅgadhara and Bhāva-miśra, viz., in the 16th century.

The work does not claim to be anything but a compilation from a large number of earlier medical works (atra granthe bhūritantrātta-sāre), including *CS, SS, AHr, Vṛnda, Tīsaṭa* and *SaS.* The topics covered are general considerations of health, illness and treatment (ch. 1); anatomy and embryology (ch. 2); measures (ch. 3); terminology (ch. 4); treatment procedures like oleation, sudation, emesis, purgation, and so on (5-12); preparation of food, articles of food, cooks and kitchen (13, 14 and 16); proper conduct during day and night and in seasons (17, 18 and 15); *materia medica* (19-40); medical uses of metals and mercury (41-43); clinical examination (44-53); curability or otherwise of diseases (54); manner of taking medicine (55); diagnosis, symptoms and treatment of specific diseases (56-147); and the treatment of diseases in general (sarvaroga-chikitsā 148).

Many Yunāni prescriptions are found included here. The employment of opium *(ahiphena)* and cinnabar *(darada)* has been mentioned. This is probably the earliest work in which Śaṁkha-drāvaka (a solvent for dissolving shells) has been referred to.

Bṛhan-nighaṇṭu-ratnākara : This is a voluminous compendium, as the name suggests, of matters of practical medical interest. (Dattarām Chaube, Veṅkaṭeshvara Press, Bombay 1891). Along with classical methods of examination and treatment, many modern methods (e.g., urine examination according to Western physicians) and drugs (e.g. tobacco) are incorporated.

The book is in six sections. Additional matter in the form of an elaborate and descriptive *materia medica* (nighaṇṭu) in two parts (7th and 8th section) has been compiled by Lālā Śālagrām. Names of drugs in Sanskrit, Latin, English and several modern Indian languages have been given.

C

Chakradattam: This work has been modelled after VṚNDA's *Siddha-Yoga,* but incorporates numerous new recipes and formulae. Besides the usual drugs, metallurgical preparations are also given here. In fact, the work seems to have been written primarily to annotate Nāgārjuna's metallurgical science (loha-śāstra), which is described as 'very obscure' (ati-gahanam).

The actual name of this work by CHAKRAPĀṆI-DATTA is *Chikitsā-saṁgraha,* but to distinguish it from another work of almost the same name (*Chikitsā-sāra-saṁgraha*) by VAṄGA-SENA, it is familiarly known as *Chakradattam* after the author's name. It is very popular in the northern regions of the country, especially in Bengal.

It is an independent work of the author, whose fame rests mainly on his commentary on *CS* (*Āyurveda dīpikā*) although he wrote other works like *Bhānumatī,* incomplete commentary on *SS, Dravya-guṇa-saṁgraha,* and a compilation of drug-details, a summary of treatments.

There is a commentary on this work, *Ratna-prabhā* by NIŚCHALA-KARA, (12th century), based on which ŚIVADĀSA-SENA wrote another gloss, called *Tātparya-chandrikā* (15th century) [*See* CHAKRAPĀṆI-DATTA.]

Chakrapāṇi-Datta: He was the author of a commentary on *CS* called *Āyurveda-dīpikā* (*Charaka-tātparya-ṭīka*), which is widely relied upon by Indian physicians. It was first published in 1892, and since then all standard editions of *CS* are equipped with this commentary. He was a native of Bengal, son of Nārāyaṇa-datta who was superviser of the royal kitchen (rasavatyādhikāri) and counsellor to the chieftain of Gauḍa, Nyapāla-deva (c. A.D. 1060). His teacher was one Nara-datta, whose identity is uncertain.

His other works are:

(1) *Chikitsā-saṁgraha* (familiarly known as *Chakradattam*), on which there is a commentary by Śivadāsa-sena *(Charaka-tattva-pradīpikā)*: this work borrows from VṚNDA'S *Siddhayoga*. It is very popular with the physicians. It seeks to present a comparative account of the two major medical traditions in India — the Ātreya (therapeutic) and the Dhānvantara (surgical). There are two commentaries *Ratna-prabhā* (Niśchala-kara's) and *Tattva-chandrikā* (Śivadāsa-sena's).

(2) *Dravya-guṇa saṁgraha,* a pharmacological work dealing with drugs prescribed in *CS, SS* and *AHr,* and with articles of food for health and hygiene.

(3) *Bhānumatī,* an incomplete commentary on *SS,* fragments of which have survived (publ. Lakshmīrāma-nidhi-granthamālā, Series I contains only Sūtra-sthānam.)

A glossary of medical terms in Ayurveda *(Āyurveda-śabda-kośá)* has been ascribed to his authorship.

Calcination of some metals has been mentioned by him, but not opium or pulse-examination.

Charaka: Regarded as one of "The Ancient Three" (Vṛddha-trayī) of Indian medicine, Charaka is the principal exponent of the medical system known as KĀYA-CHIKITSĀ (general therapeutics or internal medicine). The core-text of Āyurveda, namely, CHARAKA-SAṀHITĀ (which is also the earliest medical treatise in India) has been ascribed to him.

The identity of CHARAKA is altogether uncertain. We are not even sure if that was the personal name of the author who was principally responsible for the extant version of CHARAKA-SAṀHITĀ. It has been suggested (in *Bṛhajjātaka)* that the medical expert who travelled from village to village not only administering medicines but also teaching the medical science was called 'Charaka' (wandering physician) by the people, even as the surgeon was known as 'Dhanvantari'.

The expression 'Charaka' has been employed in this sense even in the Vedic corpus. Charakas were scholars who were affiliated to the *Kāṭhaka-Saṁhitā* and *Kṛshna-Yajurveda.* A prominent sage belonging to this Vedic branch, VAIŚAṀPĀYANA, was known as Charaka, and his disciples were also called Charakas (according to *Kāśikā-vṛtti* on Pāṇini 4,3,104.) An early Upanishad *(Bṛhadāraṇyaka,* 3,3,1) refers to the wandering scholars (Charakas) in the Madra country. Three classes of students were recognized: (1) those who, without a formal initiation, served the teacher and lived with him (mānava); (2) those who resided with the teacher after formal initiation and as regular students (antevāsi); and (3) those who, having completed a course of study under a teacher, went to other teachers for higher study for short durations (charaka). The ancient grammarian PĀṆINI has an aphorism pertaining to the words denoting the first and third classes of students (5,1,14 māṇava-charakābhyām khaṅg). Charaka in this context means a wandering scholar.

In the early Buddhist lore (e.g., *Śoṇaka-jātaka,* 5,2,427) there are references to 'wandering scholars,' getting admitted to educational institutions like Takshaśilā as 'casual students' (chārikam charantā). Takshaśilā in the north-western corner of the country, for instance, had also a medical college which was headed by an Ātreya, and where the renowned contemporary of the Buddha, JĪVAKA, the paediatrician, was a student. Charaka, during the centuries even before Christ, was thus a term signifying wandering physicians and medical teachers.

A more specific reference to a particular

physician, who was eminent both as a physician and as an author, can be gleaned from the legendary account given in *BP* (1,1). Vishṇu, in his fish incarnation resuscitated the Vedic lore from oblivion, and his attendant Ananta (Śesha, the Dragon representing Time) became proficient in the Vedic lore, which included medicine (in *Atharvaveda)*. Once Ananta chanced to descend on the earth and wander about as a 'roving ambassador' (chāra) to know how human beings fared. He was overcome by pity after seeing humanity being afflicted with numerous ailments and people dying prematurely, so he took birth as the son of a sage, Viśuddha by name, and administered medicine to the ailing folk; he also taught the medical science. He travelled continually and reached the patients wherever they were. Because he came to them as a welcome messenger (chāra), no one knew from where, he became famous as 'the wandering physician' (Charaka) [*See* BHĀVA-PRAKĀŚA].

The work thus makes him the world's first physician. But the account here curiously closes with Charaka having compiled and redacted the medical treatises (tantras) composed by the students (like AGNIVEŚA) of the sage ĀTREYA. This detail, however, agrees with the traditional account of the origin of Indian medicine, where Charaka comes only after ĀTREYA, DHANVANTARI, INDRA and the AŚVINS.

The Indian tradition places the original author of CHARAKA-SAṀHITĀ nearly a thousand years before Christ. PATAÑJALI, the great commentator on PĀNINI and the celebrated author of *Yoga-sūtra,* who lived in the second century B.C. is claimed to have redacted the original treatise of Charaka (cf. CHAKRAPĀṆI-DATTA and BHOJA among other medical authorities). But Patañjali's medical work is no longer available, and it is impossible to confirm or deny the claim. There is, however, a citation from this work by a later grammarian NĀGEŚA-BHAṬṬA *(Laghu-mañjūshā)* regarding the definition of a reliable authority *(āpta)*.

The Chinese translation of the Buddhist scripture *(Tripiṭaka)* refers to Charaka having been the court-physician of the Kushāna King Kanishka. The exact date of Kanishka is a matter of controversy, but historians are inclined to assign his reign to a period between 58 B.C. and A.D. 144. This reference would make Charaka a contemporary of the poet AŚVAGOSHA and the alchemist NĀGĀRJUNA.

The NISI Chronology Committee suggests that the original form of *CS* can be assigned to about A.D. 100. There is an alternate suggestion that the redaction of AGNIVEŚA's treatise by Charaka (now known as CHARAKA-SAṀHITĀ) is to be dated 175 B.C. The language and style of the available text supports the latter suggestion.

Considering the fact that the available text makes frequent mention of the tribes and places of northern and north-western parts of the country, it is probable that Charaka (the redactor) hailed from this region. The tribes mentioned (*CS, Chikitsā,* 30, 316), namely, Pahlava, Vāhlīka, Chīna, Śūlika, Yavana, and Śaka are all West Indian. In thosedays, thegeography of the country around the Hindukush included Vāhlīka (along the northern and western directions), Kaṁboja (along the northern and eastern directions), Gandhāra (along the southern and eastern directions) and Kapiśa (along the southern and western directions). It included also parts of Central Asia. This explains how the medical tradition expounded by Charaka had a base wider than the later confines of India.

Nothing is known about the life and career of Charaka. His father's name is given as VIŚUDDHA, a saintly scholar in the Vedic lore, in the legendary account preserved in *BP.* Who Charaka's teacher was is not known. AGNIVEŚA, whose treatise Charaka undertook to redact, stands separated from Charaka by several generations.

Besides *CS,* two works are ascribed to his authorship: a commentary on *Agniveśa-tantra* and another on *Kṛshṇa-Yajurveda,* the text of the Vedic school to which he appears to have belonged. But the ascription is unfounded.

Charaka-Saṁhitā: This is the earliest medical treatise in India that has come down to us more or less in an excellent state of preservation, although not in its original form. It is an elaborate and comprehensive manual, dealing with different aspects of disease and treatment. And it has served as the foundational work for all subsequent medical literature and practice.

The title of the work in the most authentic edition (Nirṇaya-Sāgar, Bombay, 1922) is given as *Charaka-Saṁhitā,* being the work composed by Agniveśa based on the teachings of the sage Punarvasu, as (tantra) redacted by Charaka and Dṛḍhabala. Thus four authors have been involved in the work in its extant form: Punarvasu (–Ātreya), Agniveśa, Charaka and Dṛḍhabala. Tradition makes Punarvasu-Atreya the teacher of six medical masters of whom Agniveṣa was one. Each of these six wrote a treatise, but Agniveśa's work has served as the source-book for this *Saṁhitā;* his *tantra* is no longer available in its original form. What we have now is its redaction first by Charaka and subsequently by Dṛḍhabala.

The authenticity of the ancient teaching is affirmed by the aphoristic statement at the beginning of each chapter: "Thus said the revered Ātreya" (iti ha smāha bhagavān Ātreyah). And the colophon of each chapter till *CS,* Ch. 9, reads "Thus ends ...... chapter in the work of Agniveśa as redacted by Charaka" (iti Agniveśakṛte tantre Charaka-pratisaṁskṛte), and then on "Thus ends chapter in the work of Agniveśa as redacted by Charaka, and the missing portions being supplied by Dṛḍhabala" (. . . . . aprāpte Dṛḍhabala-saṁpūrite . . .). [*See* DṚḌHABALA for his contribution.]

The nature of redaction has been indicated in the text itself while defining the expression Saṁhitā. "What has been briefly said will be elaborated, and what has been elaborated will be summarized; the redactor will thus modernize the ancient text" (*CS,* Si-sth., 12, 36). Extreme brevity and prolix elaboration are regarded as defects in a scriptural text, and they are sought to be avoided by the redactors. Modernization is with reference to the appropriate elaboration and summarization, in conformity with the needs of contemporary students.

CS is in eight divisions, or *Sthānas* and each bears a descriptive title. A *Sthāna* in its turn is divided into chapters, also bearing descriptive captions. It is an extensive work, and its volume exceeds that of its celebrated companion, Suśruta-Saṁhita, although the surgical matter is entirely left out in the former.

The eight divisions are:

(1) *Sūtra-Sthāna* (also called *Śloka-Sthāna)* in 30 chapters. This is the most important of the divisions, and deals with the entire subject-matter in a synoptical manner. There is a conventional grouping of the chapters in seven quartets (chatushka). The first (Bheshaja-chatushka) deals with general introduction to health and medicine, longevity, gruels, ointments, drugs and purgatives. The second (Svastha-vṛtta-chatushka) covers general hygiene, preventive medicine, personal health, dietetics and instructions against the suppression of natural urges. The third (Nirdeśa-chatushka) explains the four aspects of effective treatment (physician, medicine, patient and nurse) and the three goals towards which human conduct is directed (health, prosperity and spiritual welfare). The fourth (Kalpanā-chatushka) pertains to

measures, oleogenous treatment, diaphoresis, provisional treatment and physicians. The fifth one (Roga-chatushka) deals with the diseases of head and heart, swellings, abdominal ailments and major illnesses. The sixth (Yojanā-chaṭushka) deals with unfavourable human types, alternatives, ailments arising out of excesses, and illnesses caused by defilement of blood. The last one (Annapāna-chatushka) actually contains six chapters, dealing with general aetiology of ailments, views concerning taste (rasa), food and drink, dietetics, 'seats' of life. The last chapter contains an analytical content of the entire book.

(2) *Nidāna-Sthāna* (8 chapters) deals with general pathology of eight major diseases: fevers (jvara), haemorrhage (raktapitta), tumours (gulma), urinary ailments (prameha), skin troubles including leprosy (kushṭha), pthisis (śosha), mental aberrations (unmāda) and epilepsy (apasmāra). Each chapter furnishes details concerning the disease-types, causation and manifestation of diseases, diagnostic aids, and treatment procedures. Helpful hints are given to the attending physician.

(3) *Vimāna-Sthāna* (8 chapters) deals with miscellaneous matter: chemistry and physiology of rasa (taste), three major divisions of the stomach, epidemics and infectious ailments, the three diagnostic procedures (observation, inference and testimony), the circulatory, digestive and evacuatory functions, varieties of disturbances in body and mind together with their prognostic assessment, types of patients, varieties of bodily parasites (krimi), and matters pertaining to medical education.

(4) *Śārīra-Sthāna* (8 chapters) deals with general human constitution, progeny, pregnancy, foetal development, growth, physiological framework, life and death. There are philosophical discussions concerning man and the environment. It also enumerates the anatomical parts of the body, and in the last chapter we find an account of midwifery.

(5) *Indriya-Sthāna* (12 chapters) deals mainly with symptomatological diagnosis and prognosis. The major part of the division is devoted to the ascertainment of the approach of death by various signs and symptoms.

(6) *Chikitsā-Sthāna* (30 chapters) is the most valuable division for the practising physician as it contains numerous drug-formulae and prescriptions for long and healthy life. It includes details concerning rejuvenation (rasāyana) and virilification (vājīkaraṇa).

Treatment of diseases like fever, tumour, diabetes, phthisis, insanity, epilepsy, abdominal ailments, piles, diarrhoea, anaemia, hiccough, asthma, vomiting, erysipelas, abnormal thirst, delirium, diseases of bladder, heart and head, nervous ailments, leprosy and diseases of women, are dealt with here.

(7) *Kalpa-Sthāna* (12 chapters) is the division that deals with drugs (especially for emesis and purgation), formulae, and pharmacy.

(8) *Siddhi-Sthāna* (12 chapters) deals with the methods of effective treatment, especially, with the classical Pañcha-Karma.

Although the work refers to the eight-fold medicine (Ashṭāṅga-Āyurveda), it principally deals with only one branch, viz., Kāya-Chikitsā. It casually deals with the other branches, except major surgery (Śalya) which is altogether excluded.

The work reveals the author's extensive acquaintance with plant, mineral and animal resources for treatment of diseases. There is a clear preference for drugs of vegetable extraction. [See OSHADHI].

The style of the work is direct and engaging; the language has close links with the *brāhmaṇa* passages of the Vedic Corpus. There are long prose passages as well as short sentences together with strings of verses. Two philosophical systems Sāṁkhya and Nyāya are heavily relied upon (*CS, Śā,* I and VI, 4,4,12). The Sāṁkhya that we find in this work is more ancient than the one found in Īśvara-Kṛshṇa's *Sāṁkhya-Kārikā*. The Yoga system also is referred to, but the Yoga advocated here is slightly different from Patañjali's (*CS, Sa,* 5, II-26). The Veda is accepted as reliable authority (āptāgama), but not making much of it. Good conduct is advocated as the necessary precondition for health. While the general attitude is rational and treatment prescribed is largely drug-oriented, there is also a suggestion for reinforcement by rituals and worship. Some divinities (Indra, Brahmā, Vishṇu, Lakshmī, Viśvakarmā and Vṛsha-dhvaja or Śiva) are also mentioned, but not with any importance attached to them. Vishṇu-sahasra-nāma has, however, been commended as a cure for fevers (*CS,* Ch. 3, 312).

The work comprehends mainly all the lessons given by Punarvasu-Ātreya to Agniveśa and others in assemblies of sages who were medical authorities (e.g., *CS, Sū,* 25, 1-29 and 26, 3-9). The work mentions as many as 60 earlier medical authorities; many of them are well-known sages like Vaśishṭha, Jamadagni, Bhṛgu and Vaṁadeva; but there are some who are little known, like Kāpya, Śaraloma, Vaḍiśa and Hiraṇyāksha. The medical views of many of these sages are also recorded.

The work elaborately discusses the physiology of the three Doshas, human anatomy, diagnosis and prognosis of diseases, foetal growth during the months, and medical education.

His account of anatomy, however, is elementary, the total number of bones (including teeth) being 360, and muscles are regarded as merely fleshy masses. The structures of the heart and brain appear to be little understood; and the lungs are not associated with respiration.

During the foetal growth, limbs are said to be initially differentiated in the fourth month; awareness is structured in the fifth and intelligence emerges as an organismic function in the sixth.

His *materia medica* is extensive with 341 drugs of vegetable origin, 177 drugs of animal origin and 64 drugs of mineral and metallic origin. He has also classified the vegetable drugs according to the parts of the plants utilized: roots of 16 plants, fruits of 19 plants and juice of three barks are of medicinal value. He has divided plants into 50 groups, each having over 10 plants (*CS, Sū, Sth.,* 1,4).

"Charaka was a person of great culture and intellect and prepared his work for the general guidance of the humanity in the ways of life and health." And in this sense, *CS* is said to be "a far more interesting work" than *SS*.

There are numerous commentaries on this work, many of which however, are not extant. The most celebrated and frequently printed commentary is by CHAKRAPĀṆI-DATTA, known as ĀYURVEDA-DĪPIKĀ (Or *Charaka-tātparya-ṭīkā*). Among other commentaries which were well-known once but have since been neglected, lost or mutilated are, BHAṬṬĀRA-HARICHANDRA'S *Charaka-nyāsa* (fragmentary MSS, first three chapters of *CS,* Sū., GOML, No. 13092, about 6th century), JAIJJAṬA'S *Nirantara-pada-vyākhyā* (about A.D. 875), ŚIVADĀSA-SENA'S *Charaka-tattva-pradīpikā* (around A.D. 1460) and SVĀMI-KUMĀRA'S *Pañjikā* or *Pañchikā* (GOML, vol.23, No. 13091, incomplete) merit mention. References to several other commentaries that have been irretrievably lost are available: they are by Patañjali, Īśāna-deva, Vyāpya-Chandra, Vakula, Nara-datta, Guṇākara, Govardhana, Bhīma-datta, Jina-dāsa, Jaya-nandi and Īśvara-sena. Among the more recent commentaries are NARASIṀHA KAVIRĀJA'S

Charaka-tattva-prakāśa, Kaustubha, YOGENDRANĀTHA SEN'S *Charakopaskara* (incomplete) and GANGĀDHARA-KAVIRATNA'S *Jalpa-kalpa-taru.*

The work had been translated into Persian and later into Arabic by the 8th century (mentioned in *Fihrst* A.D. 987). al-Beruni, who incidentally held that Charaka was the most ancient of Indian medical writers, relied on the Arabic translation of *CS* by Ali-ibn-Zain of Tarbistan. *Sharaka Indianus* is to be found in the Latin translation of Rhazes (b. A.D. 680) and Avicenna.

Among the early editions of *CS*, prominent ones are by Jībānanda Vidyāsāgara (Calcutta 1877), Gaṅgādhara-Kaviratna (Berhampur 1879), Harinātha Viśārada (1895) and Vāman Keshava Dātār (Nirṅaya-sāgar, Bombay 1922). The work was translated into English by A.C. Kaviratna in 1920 (Calcutta). A six-volume edition of the text with transl. into English, Gujarāthi and Hindī was brought out in 1949 (Jāmnagar, Gujarat Āyurvedic Society).

Charakopaskara: An incomplete but valuable gloss on *CS* by Yogīndranāth-Sen (1871-1918), a leading physician of Bengal. The work was designed to help the student in understanding *CS* aright.

Chikitsā-kalikā: This is a text book by TĪSATA (c. A.D.500, mainly in the nature of a compendium of well-known formulae (yoga).

The work is in 400 elegant verses (vṛtta-śataiś chaturbhih) dealing with general therapeutics (kāya-chikitsā). There are accounts of other branches of medicine, like surgery, bhūta-vidyā and rejuvenation, but they are exceedingly brief. Even the anatomical information is scanty and cursory. The formulae are extracted from earlier authorities like Bhela, Kāśyapa and Śukra.

It reminds one of *Nāvanītaka* but is more elaborate. The prescriptions are mostly from plants and trees.

There is a gloss (*vivṛti*) on this work by the author's son CHANDRAṬA. The work has been quoted in *Vīrasiṁhāvaloka* (1383). [*See* TĪSAṬA]

Chinese Medicine: Medicine in China is said to have originated with two patriarchs: Shen-nung (2757 B.C., author of the first *Materia Medica* in the world) and Huang-ti (2697 B.C., author of the *Canon of Medicine*). Both are legendary heroes, and Chinese medicine really dates from about 205 B.C., when the earliest physician, Chang-Chung-K'ung, lived and practised. He wrote a treatise on fevers, their diagnosis, clinical examination, symptomatology, course, management and treatment. Contemporaneous with him was the first surgeon in China, Hua-tu, who employed anaesthesia. These two may be described as the Charaka and Suśruta of China.

The foundation on which the entire Chinese medicine rested and developed is the Taoist doctrine of the twin forces of 'Yin' and 'Yang', which constitute and govern the entire creation. Formulated around 300 B.C., the doctrine spoke of the two forces as curiously antagonistic and complementary. 'Yin', representing 'Earth', is dark, weak, feminine and passive; it corresponds with the Moon. 'Yang' on the other hand, represents 'Heaven' and corresponds with the Sun; it is light, strong, masculine and active. Human body, being a miniature model of the universe, not only accommodates these two fundamental forces, but is subject to them.

Balance between the twin forces means health, and its disruption can occur owing to the momentary weakening of one of the five elements that enter into the constitution of the body: water, fire, wood, metal and earth. There are five organs intimately related to the five elements: kidney, heart, liver, lungs and spleen, in order. The disruption of the balance is located principally in one or other of these five organs.

The identification of the organ in which the disturbance has occurred is made possible by examining the pulse. Pulse-examination is an important detail in Chinese medicine. The other examinations of colours, viscera, bowel and bodily appearance follow closely the pulse-examination. Each hand has three sets of pulses connected with the organs; and each pulse in its turn has an outer and an inner pulselet, the twelve pulses being thus connected with the entire body.

The normal rate of pulse beats was considered to be four, viz., time taken for the physician to complete an act of breathing (one inhalation and one exhalation). The pulses are three in number on each hand, technically designated as 'inch', 'bar', and 'cubit'. As they are felt by the physician with light touch or with some pressure, they indicate the condition of the twelve major parts of the body wherein disturbances are likely to occur. As the physician feels the pulse, he watches whether the pulse is superficial or deep, even or irregular, gentle or frisky.

The pulse-examination is essentially of diagnostic value: it gives the physician the clue as regards the part of the body in which the disease has originated, and also whether it is the 'Yin' or 'Yang' that is disturbed. It can also be a prognostic aid; it will enable the physician to assess the curability or otherwise of the ailment. Further, the line of treatment that the physician must prescribe is also indicated.

The aim of the treatment would be to restore the natural balance between the two fundamental forces 'Yin' and 'Yang'. The treatment is divided into two major kinds : preventive and curative. The former is given the greater importance : diseases are prevented (or health is maintained) by the individual being harmoniously adjusted to nature, viz., following the Tao. A simple life, eschewing excesses and observing the laws of nature, are advocated. Treatment of the 'spirit' (*Ch'i*) which is thereby vouchsafed is the essence of preventive medicine.

The food that we eat and the habits that we cultivate regarding it can constitute a mode of treatment that nourishes the physical body. Proper diet and right habits of eating can treat the ailments without any medicine. Food, which like the body is made up of the five elements, is distinguished by five tastes: sweet, sour, pungent, bitter and salty. Each taste is a mode of nourishment. The proper diet balances all the tastes.

The treatment procedure that is curative in character relies on drugs. Each drug is regarded as a judicious mixture of the two forces 'Yin' and 'Yang', so that the disturbed balance between them in the body (which the disease in fact means) is corrected and restored. Herbal drugs also dominate Chinese medicine. The first *Materia Medica* which was composed around 2000 B.C., was later expanded to include 400 kinds of herbs. In the 16th century, it came to contain 8000 prescriptions with 2000 drugs, the majority of which was from the vegetable kingdom. During the early part of the 19th century, *The Names and Virtues of Plants* ran into 60 volumes!

The basic idea in treatment is that most of the illnesses are caused by an imbalance between 'Yin' and 'Yang' reflected in the disharmony of the five elements known as 'dyscrasia', owing to the external influences of weather and season (in terms of wind, fire, heat, cold, dryness or humidity) or by internal factors (joy, anger, desire, surprise, grief, fear or worry).The treatment is directed towards restoration of the balance. Herbs, being most in line with the Tao, are regarded as most effective in correcting the 'dyscrasia' of the elements.

An alternate line of treatment is 'acupuncture', which has made Chinese medicine famous all over the world. Also based on the theory of the interaction of the twin principles of 'Yin' and 'Yang', this system works on the rather unusual conception of surface anatomy.

The two forces are unequally distributed in the physical body, and the strife between the parts in which 'Yang' is superfluous, and the parts in which 'Yin' is deficient manifests itself as disease. The two forces together with the superfluity or deficiency are carried to different parts of the body along 12 (or 14, according to some) channels which distribute blood and breath throughout the body. The channels are connected with all the vital organs. The surface anatomy accepted by the advocates of acupuncture recognizes 365 (or 349 in another account) vital spots distributed all over the body, especially in the head and the extremities, and it is at these spots that the channels (which are deep within the musculature) surface.

Breath and blood, in a healthy person, would flow evenly within the channels, and the vital spots would reflect this smooth flow. Pulse-examination reveals this state of affairs as also any disturbances in the flow. When the vital forces that course through the channels become superfluous or abundant, tension is felt at the spots in the shape of blocks. When they become deficient, the spots reveal a certain slackness. Puncturing the chosen spots would rectify the error. The blocks are supposed to be caused by the accumulation of foul breath at these junctures; puncturing in that case would help the excess air to escape, thus relieving the tension of the breath. When the flow is deficient, puncturing would energize and stimulate. In either case, the disturbed coordination of 'Yin' and 'Yang' is corrected.

Proper puncturing (also called 'needling') is accomplished by special needles made of gold, silver, copper or steel. There is a mention of nine different kinds of needles in use. The kind of needle to be used, choice of the spots to be punctured, the discovery of the deficiency of 'Yin' or the superfluity of 'Yang', the amount of pressure to be exerted while needling, the direction in which the needle should slant (along the vital flow or against it) and so on are some of the complex aspects of this art of healing.

All types of diseases are claimed to be treated and healed by acupuncture. The *Canon of Medicine* (*Nei-Ching-su-Wen*) which Huang-ti is said to have written around 2690 B.C., gives a detailed account of the ailments that are sought to be cured by acupuncture. It also contains a comprehensive account of the art of acupuncture, and of its theoretical foundation ('Yin' and 'Yang').

The same author, who is regarded as the 'Father of Chinese medicine', also prescribes another treatment-procedure to be employed along with acupuncture. This is known as 'moxibustion' (also called 'Moxa'), after the material from the plant *moxa* (*Artemisia vulgaris*) that constitutes the main therapeutic ingredient. The leaves of this plant are dried and powdered and rolled into the shape of cigarettes or cones. The spot on the skin is chosen precisely as in acupuncture, and the cigarette or cone is placed in it vertically and is lighted; the cigarette is allowed to burn for a specified period (up to 30 min.), and the heat is said to draw off the ailing condition that is deep within the channels that carry the 'Yin' and 'Yang' forces. The heat that is principally employed here for the therapeutic purpose shares the property of 'Yang' (masculine and active force). It will, therefore, correct the superfluity of 'Yin'. The cigarettes are sometimes allowed to burn long enough to cause a blister on the spot.

The technique of moxibustion is said to be older than acupuncture, and Confucius himself is supposed to have evolved this technique. However, there are conditions in which both are employed; and these are explained in great detail in the classic *Nei-Ching*. Both the techniques are based on the original Taoist idea of twin-forces ('Yin' and 'Yang').

Although surgery began in China in the distant past, it did not make a headway; and its appeal gradually weakened, probably because of the doctrinal emphasis on non-interference with nature. Therefore, the anatomical knowledge of the ancient Chinese was also limited. But the exceedingly rich pharmacopoeia that they developed and the highly sophisticated techniques of acupuncture and moxibustion that they evolved and perfected more than compensated for this lacuna.

One can readily recognize the numerous correspondences that exist between Chinese and Indian medicine. The basic ideas appear to be almost identical: the individual being a miniature model of the universe, the elemental constitution of the organism, the life-force working itself through the individual, the concept of strategic spots in the body, the need for living in close conformity with nature, the medicinal value of food, the twin energy-strands, the emphasis on restoration of balance as the physician's task, the importance attached to personal hygiene and prophylaxis, the reliance on herbal drugs, and the unfavourable outlook on surgery.

It has recently been discovered that acupuncture also was practised in ancient India. Massaging (aṅga-mardana) was another art that was developed as auxiliary to medicine both in China and India. Likewise the practice of modulated breathing (prānāyāma) prescribed in Yoga as well as Āyurveda was also advocated in China as early as 2000 B.C.

It was only in China and India that medicine was provided with a sound philosophical foundation, and an attempt was made to relate the therapeutic practices with theoretical constructs.

D

Ḍalhaṇa: Ḍalhaṇa or Ḍallaṇa is the author of the celebrated and complete commentary on *SS*, known as *Nibandha-saṁgraha.*

He hailed from the village Aṅkolā near Mathurā, and was the son of the physician BHARATA-PĀLA; he was patronized by a feudatory of the King of Mathurā, SAHAPĀLA, who governed the area called Bhādānaka.

His date is uncertain, but he probably belongs to the 10th century A.D. He does not quote Chkp's commentary on *SS (Bhānumatī),* but Chkp. criticizes the views of Ḍalhaṇa. He must, therefore, be earlier than Chkp (A.D. 1060)

His commentary is lucid and elaborate, especially meant to help the students. He quotes from earlier commentaries on *SS,* viz., by BHOJA, JAIJJAṬA GAYADĀSA, BHĀSKARA, (Pañjikā) and BRAHMADEVA *(Ṭippaṇa),* from whom he has derived much help. This commentary has a gloss by ARUṆADATTA, known as *Sarvāṅga-Sundarī.* [*See* SUŚRUTA-SAṀHITĀ].

Dhanvantari: Regarded as the original exponent of Indian medicine, Dhanvantari has many myths and legends woven around him. He emerged with the pot of ambrosia (symbolic of medicine) in his hand from the ocean when it was churned by the contesting gods and demons. He is viewed as the very incarnation of Vishṇu (cf., *Mahābhārata, Ādi,* 1140; *Rāmāyaṇa,* I, 45, 32; *Bhāgavata,* 8, 8, 34; *Harivaṁśa,* 29, 1523; *Vishṇu-purāṇā,* 4,8,4). He is said to have recovered ambrosia which had been lost, and thus obtained a share in sacrifices (yajñabhuj).

Legends make him reappear as Divodāsa, the prince of Banaras (Kāśirājā), in the family of Āyus. According to *SS*, Dhanvantari, Divodāsa and Kāśirāja are names of the same person who is "the first god and who freed the other gods from old age, disease and death" (Dhanvantarir ādidevo jarā-rujā-mṛtyu-haro'marāṇām), and who in his Himālayan retreat taught surgery to Suśruta and other sages. BP explains that Dhanvantari appeared on earth in Banaras in the princely family of Bāhuja and became known as Divodāsa, that he wandered about as a mendicant even during his early years, and that Brahmā persuaded him to accept the crown of Banaras (Kāśirāja). However, there are accounts which make Dhanvantari the son of Kāśirāja, and Kāśirāja the grandson of Dhanvantari. There may thus be more than one Dhanvantari, the earliest of whom was called Āyus (who was the son of Purūravas). The lineage preserved in *Vishṇu-purāṇa* (4,8) is: Purūravas-Āyus-Kshatravṛdha-Kāśa-Kāśirāja (name, not 'king of Kāśī') — Dīrghatamas (Dīrgatapas in *Harivaṁśa)* — Dhanvantari-Ketumāna-Divodāsa.

Dhanvantari is not mentioned in *RV*, but Divodāsa figures prominently (e.g., 1,116,18; 6,16,5; 6,31,4). And Divodāsa is here intimately associated with the sage Bhāradvāja, who in turn is associated with the Aśvins, Agni, and Indra. Śāṅkhāyana-gṛhya-sūtra (2,14) connects Dhanvantari with Bhāradvāja. In the traditional account of the origin of Indian medicine, Dhanvantari learnt medicine from Bhāradvāja, who in turn was taught by Indra, and he by the Aśvins (although BP would make Dhanvantari the direct disciple of Indra (adhītya chāyusho vedam Indrād Dhanvantarih purā); Ātreya and Bhāradvāja, according to this work, were Indra's disciples on different occasions, and Ātreya taught Bhāradvāja. Chakrapāṇi would identify Ātreya with Bhāradvāja. [*See* ĀTREYA].

A work of recent origin but enshrining an old legend, also makes Bhāradvāja teach Dhanvantari who had been born as an 'aṁbashṭa' (born of a Brahmin father, the sage Gālava, and a *vaiśya* girl Vīrabhadrā), and as the progenitor of the Vaidya caste *(Aṁbashṭāchāra-chandrikā).*

Dhanvantari appears to have been an actual historical person, although his precise identity is hard to be ascertained. He taught surgery (Śalyāṅga), one of the eight divisions of Ayurveda, at the instance of Suśruta, to a group of sages among whom Suśruta was the foremost. Ḍalhaṇa enumerates 12 of his disciples: Aupadhenava, Vaitaraṇa, Aurabhra, Paushkalāvata, Karavīrya Gopura-rakshita, Suśruta, Bhoja, Nimi, Kaṅkāyana, Gārgya, and Gālava (*NS* I, I). The names of Nimi, Kaṅkāyana, Gārgya and Suśruta and their formulae are mentioned in the *Bower Mss (Nāvanītaka),* where Suśruta appears as the student of 'ascetic (*muni*) Kāśirāja'. Of the names of masters mentioned here, Gārgya figures also as a student of Ātreya (*CS,* 11).

The disciples of Dhanvantari are said to have compiled their own medical treatises. While Suśruta's is only the one that has come down (*See* SUŚRUTA-SAṀHITĀ), we have references to the treatises of others; some of them have also been quoted, as, e.g. PAUSHKALĀVATA's views in *Āyurveda-dīpikā,* (Chkp on *CS*), *Bhānumatī* (Chkp on *SS*); *Tattva-Chandrikā;* Karavīrya's prescriptions in *NS* and *VyMk;* Gopurakshita in *NS,* and *Tattva-Chandrikā,* Vaitaraṇa's formulae in the same works as also in Chakra-datta (where Vaitaraṇa-Vasti, an enema, is referred to).

Although Dhanvantari is credited with the division of Ayurveda into eight branches (aṅgas) (cf., *Vishṇu-purāṇa,* 4,8,4), he as well as his disciples are associated mainly with surgery. That is why the tradition of surgery in India is known as 'Dhānvantara-saṁpradāya' to distinguish it from the tradition of therapeutics known as 'Ātreya-sampradāya.' Even Charaka refers to surgeons as 'dhānvantarīyah' (*CS, Chik.Sth.* 5, 'tatra dhānvantarīyāṇāṃ adhikārah kriyā-vidhau).

But Dhanvantari is regarded as the patron-god of all branches of medicine. Indeed, according to *Garuḍa-purāṇa,* (142, 5-6) he taught Suśruta all the eight branches of Āyurveda (āyurvedam athāṣṭhāṅgam Suśrutāya cha uktavān), although Suśruta's name is especially associated with one of them (śalya, surgery).

Dhanvantari is not credited with any medical treatise of his own, in the early accounts. *Brahma-vaivarta-purāṇa,* where Dhanvantari, Divodāsa, and Kāśirāja are regarded as different persons, ascribes *Chikitsā-tattva-vijñāna* to Dhanvantari; the work, however, has not come down to us. There is a voluminous glossary and *materia medica* in nine sections known as *Dhanvantari-nighaṇṭu;* but it is a compilation which is probably contemporaneous with the famous *Amara-kosha* (c. A.D. 100). There are a few other works (like *Roga-nidāna, Chikitsā-sāra-saṁgraha,* and *Vaidyaka-bhāskarodaya)* which are ascribed to Dhanvantari, but the ascription is obviously spurious.

There are numerous preparations which are ascribed to him, and many of them are quite ancient: Dhānvantara-ghṛta, Pāśupata-rasa, Mṛtyuñjaya-lauha, Rasa-rājendra, Rasābhra-guggulu, Aśvagandhādi-taila, and Dhānvantara-guṭikā (a guggulu pill with 32 ingredients).

Dhanvantari-Nighaṇṭu: Also known as *Dravyāvalī,* it is ascribed to Dhanvantari, who is obviously not the celebrated Divodāsa who was the teacher of Suśruta. The composition of this work is earlier than 1150 (when the poet Maṅkha knew it), and even prior to the compilation of the lexicon *Amara-Kosha* (1st cent. A.D.). It is the most ancient of the medical glossaries that are available.

The original work is said to have been in three recensions; the present version which may have been based on one of them, is in six sections (vargas) and deals with 373 medicinal substances (dravyas), their names, synonyms, and brief description of properties being given.

The work which claims to be "like the third eye" (tṛtīyam api lochanam) for the practising physician, is extensively relied upon, despite several more comprehensive glossaries that have been compiled subsequently. [*See* NIGHAṆṬU]

Dravya-dīpikā: A gloss over Trimalla-bhaṭṭa's *Dravya-guṇa-śataka* prepared by KṚSHṆA-DATTA-MIŚRA, son of ŚIVA-DATTA-MIŚRA of the Karpūriya clan (author of *Nānārthaushadhi-kōsha*). [*See* ŚIVA-KOSHA]. The author has sought to bridge the gap between the classical pharmacological theories and their practical utility. He advances a fresh outlook on substances, qualities, taste, etc.

Dravya-guṇa-saṁgraha: This is an early *materia medica*, compiled by CHAKRAPĀṆI-DATTA (around A.D. 1060), mainly following *CS* and *SS.* The major part of it deals with articles of diet for the patient, but no medicinal substances have been described therein.

The topics that are dealt with here are foodgrains, meat, vegetables, salts, fruits, water, milk, oils, sugar-cane products (ikshu-vikṛti), wines and liquor, cooked rice (kṛtānna), prescriptions concerning food (āhāra-vidhi), and articles of food that have to be taken after medicament (anupāna). Substances that are of food value (āhāra-dravya) are primarily nourishment-oriented (rasa-pradhāna), while articles of medicinal value (aushadha-dravya) are predominantly potency-oriented (vīrya-pradhāna). [*See* NIGHAṆṬU].

Dravya-guṇa-saṁgraha: A pharmacological work prepared by *Chkp* (11th century) giving mainly details about the health value of the articles of food. The author claims that he has consulted numerous treatises and drawn their essential points (*tantrānām sāram ākṛshya*) (Bombay 1925, with comm. by Jvālā-prasād Miśra).

The work begins with an account of the taste, property, potency, etc., of the drugs, which have been dealt with in 15 sections: cereals, meat, vegetables, salts, etc.; fruits, drinks, milk, oils, sugar-cane, etc.; fermented drinks, preparations of food, eatables, principles to be followed while eating, anupāna, and miscellaneous.

Dravya-guṇa-śataka: A manual in 102 verses, dealing with pharmacology, it is compiled by TRIMALLA-BHAṬṬA, author of *Yoga-taraṅginī,* and a Telugu Brahmin who resided at Vārāṇasī. One of the MSS is dated A.D. 1665 (samvat 1725). The work became popular all over the country (Khemraj Sri Krishnadas, Bombay 1896).

The work, which follows *Bhāva-prakāśa* and *Madana-vinoda*, is in 15 sections. The opening verse (2) deals with the effect of the six tastes on the *doshas.* Following this are treated: water, milk and its products, cereals, meat, vegetables, sugarcane and honey, oils, fruits, spices, prepared food, fermented liquors (sandhāna), alcoholic drinks (madya), massage and bath, betel-chewing, and metals. Among metals, zinc (yaśada) and lead (nāga) are not referred to.

Dravya-guṇa-śata-ślokī: This is a medical glossary (also known as *Pathyāpathya-nighaṇṭu*), prepared by TRIMALLA-BHAṬṬA (between A.D. 1383 and 1479). Its 100 verses arranged in 14 sections (vargas) deal with different varieties of water, milk, grains, meat, plant-products (leaves, flowers, roots and fruits), sugar-cane, oils, honey, grapes, ginger, etc., boiled rice, wines and liquor, cosmetics and betel-leaves. The emphasis is on dietetics. [*See* NIGHAṆṬU]

Dravyāvalī: A pharmacological lexicon that has got mixed up in course of time with *Dhanvantari-nighaṇṭu.* The introductory verses of the latter work claim *Dravyāvalī* to be the title of the entire work. There is also a mention in it that *Dravyāvalī* ascertained for the benefit of scholarly physicians the names of 373 drugs (7,4). "Without acquaintance with such a work, the physician would become a laughing stock. .... Should he have this work, it is like having a third eye." (15)

Dhanvantari-nighaṇṭu assumed its present form over at least two or three centuries. Actually, it consists of two distinct works, one of which is *Dravyāvalī*, a list of drugs, described through synonyms. Later, there was another work which gave also the qualities and actions of each of these drugs; but the name of this work has not survived. The composite work, which became celebrated as *Dhanvantari-nighaṇṭu* (bearing however no relationship to Dhanvantari), got its present form during 10th to 13th centuries of the Christian era. [*See* DHANVANTARI-NIGHAṆṬU.]

In some of the MSS obtained from Mahārāshtra, the authorship of *Dravyāvalī* has been ascribed to MAHENDRA-BHOGIKA, son of KṚSHṆA-BHOGIKA, a resident of Sthāṇeśvara.

Dṛḍhabala: Dṛḍhabala is a redactor of *CS*, who also supplied the missing portions. It is not known if Charaka had redacted the entire *Agniveśa-Tantra*; if he had, it must not have survived in its entirety by the time the work was begun by Dṛḍhabala, who claims that the last 41 chapters were contributed by himself: 17 chapters of *Chikitsā-sthāna* and the entire divisions of *Kalpa-sthāna* and *Siddhi-shtāna,* consisting of 24 chapters (*CS, Chi.Sthāna* 30, 289 and 290) NS edition. And the colophons from *Chi. Sthāna* 9 in *CS* till the end have the words, "Thus ends the chapter in the *tantra* of Agniveśa as redacted by Charaka and the missing portions being supplied by Dṛḍhabala" (iti Agniveśa-kṛte tantre Charaka-pratisaṁskṛte aprāpte Dṛḍhabala-pūrite).

It is difficult to ascertain which 17 of the 30 chapters in *Chikitsa-sthāna* are his contributions. It is probable that the last 17 chapters of this division together with the subsequent two divisions had been lost. This amounts to about one-third of the whole work. Dṛḍhabala probably recast the entire text, and his redaction came to be known as 'Kashmir recension' (*kāśmīra-pāṭha*)

Dṛḍhabala was the son of Kapila-bala, himself a physician, and an inhabitant of Pañchanada-pura ("the town which has five rivers"). This town has been identified as Pañjor or Pañchapanor ('pañchanīra'?, 'five canals') in Kāshmīr near the confluence of Zhelum (Vitastā) and Indus (Sindhū), a few miles north of Śrīnagar.

His date is uncertain; but he has been assigned to the latter part of the third or the early part of the fourth century.

E

Egyptian Medicine: Egyptian medicine, which has many close correspondences with Indian medicine, developed in the period commencing about 3500 B.C. and continued to play an important role till 332 B.C., when the Macedonean adventurer, Alexander, overran the country and conquered it. Our knowledge of this system of medicine is principally derived from several ancient medical *papyri* (paper MSS), now named after their discoverers (like *The Ebers Papyrus, The Edwin-Smith p., The Hearst p.*, and *The Chester-Beatty p.*) or the places in which their study was undertaken (like *The London p.*, and *The Berlin p.*), and also from the Greek and Roman references to the Egyptian medical practices.

Patronized by the ruling Pharaohs and cultivated by the powerful priests, medicine developed within the framework of royalty and religion. The combination of prescriptive medicine with exorcism, magical spells and incantations was a conspicuous feature. But the concern for prolongation of life, especially in the royal household and among the nobility, and the elimination of incapacitating ailments among the soldiers and the working classes were chief motivations for the discovery and preparation of numerous drugs (about 700) from vegetable, animal and mineral sources.

The standard practices of embalming and mummification led to a fairly comprehensive knowledge of human anatomy and physiology. The interior of the human cadaver was thoroughly explored, and various secretions within the body were precisely identified. There was need to clear the body cavities of their contents, to remove the diaphragm, abdominal viscera and other parts of the body which were liable to interfere with the preservation of the form of the dead person, to extricate and remove the brain dexterously from the bony box, to leave intact and in their places the heart, the eyes and the tongue, as religious rituals required during these practices. This is a great spur to the empirical understanding of the structure and functions of the human body. ATHOTIS, a prince of the first-dynasty (about 3400 B.C.), is credited with a book on anatomy.

The priests who specialized in magic and theurgy also developed therapeutics and surgery; temples (especially in Memphis, Thebes and Sais) housed medical schools. Diseases were normally fought by a team of priests, physicians and magicians. However, in due course, medical practitioners freed themselves from the hold of religious ideas to a considerable extent, and set out to specialize in ophthalmology, dentistry, gynaecology, general medicine and surgery (as was noticed by the Greek traveller Herodotus). Clinical examination also became sophisticated and standardized. Physicians were organized in guilds.

There is one *papyrus* ('*The Edwin-Smith p.*'), the contents of which are almost exclusively matters of surgery in connection with wounds, tumours, abscesses, hernia, jaw-dislocations, bone-fractures and so on. Elaborate bandages with splints, linen and oil, and ointments have been described. Many elementary surgical procedures have been mentioned, as also the diagnostic and prognostic considerations that are involved in surgical operations.

Egyptian medicine recognized the need to understand the nature of the internal fluids, secretions and waste-products before the cure for a disease is effected. The fluids as well as air are circulated in the body through a network of arteries (called metu), which can become hard, get constricted, or lose efficiency — thus causing disease. While circulating the fluids and air throughout the body, the disturbed arteries communicate disease also to the associated organs. The drug that is administered by the physician travels through the same arteries and reaches the relevant organs, effecting remedial changes in them.

Among the vegetable drugs employed by the Egyptians are included onion, garlic, castor oil, mustard, linseed, saffron and aloes. The medicinal uses of resins, opium, metallic salts, iron, nitrate of potash, mercury, honey, and lime were known to the Egyptian physicians. Precious stones were powdered and administered as drugs. *The Ebers papyrus* (c. 1600 B.C.) deals with the preparations of medicines.

Heart was regarded as the main organ, as the physician was required to understand "The movements of the heart" in different parts of the body by feeling them with his fingers. It would appear that pulse-examination was a standard procedure in diagnosis, as it was in Chinese medicine. Although it is not certain that Egyptians, were aware of the phenomenon of blood-circulation or its relation to heart, they held that heart was the organ (in collaboration with the stomach) where blood was prepared from the food that is eaten.

Egyptian medicine was highly appreciated in Greece, and it had an enormous impact, albeit indirect, on the development of European medicine. The Greek *materia medica* and the doctrine of humours can both be traced to Egyptian sources. In fact, the historians of medicine like Ebell have viewed Greek medicine as a continuation and development of Egyptian medicine.

G

Gada-Nigraha: This is a comprehensive treatise on all branches of medicine by SOḌHALA, who belonged to Gujarat, and was probably a contemporary of VAṄGASENA (c. A.D. 1119). The author is described as a physician of Vatsa-gotra, son of Vaidya-nandana (which perhaps was not his actual name), a Gurjara Brāhmin of Roykabal sect, and a student of SAṀGHADAYĀLU.

The work is in ten sections (khaṇḍa), the first of which (called 'Prayoga-khaṇḍa') incorporates numerous (more than 585) well tried remedies (powders, pills, pastes, medicated ghees, oils, etc.). The next eight sections deal with the eight classical branches of Āyurveda; the last section pertains to the five treatment – procedures (pañchakarma).

The author appears to have had an acquaintance with *MN* and *Vṛnda*, but not with *Chakradattam* (the celebrity of which probably had not by then spread to the western regions). (ed. by Y.T. Āchārya, Bombay, 1911 and 1915).

Gayadāsa: He is the author of an incomplete commentary on *SŚ*, called *Nyāya-Chandrikā* familiarly, *Chandrikā* or *Bṛhat-pañjikā* or *Suśruta-pañjikā* (*Pañjikā*), which is quoted by ḌALHAṆA frequently. His commentary on *CS* also is fragmentary. He refers to *SS* as 'śalya-tantra', a work on surgery.

He was the court-physician of some king of the Pāla dynasty in Bengal (Gauḍeśvarāntaraṅga, *Ratna-prabhā)*.

He is placed in the 10th century. [*See* SUŚRUTA-SAṀHITĀ].

Greek theory of humours: The concept of doshas in Indian medicine is often likened to the Greek theory of 'humours'. While there are ideas that are common or very similar, there are also differences which are fundamental. An understanding of the Greek theory would clear misunderstandings.

Although the theory is usually associated with Hippocrates of Cos (460 – 377 B.C.), it dates back to the philosophical speculations of Anaximander (c. 611 B.C.) and the medical suppositions of Empedocles of Arringentum (504-433 B.C.), and the latter belonged to one of the three pre-Hippocratic medical schools in Greece, namely, the Sicilian school of Croton, founded by the celebrated Pythagoras in 532 B.C. He held that all things in the world including the human body were basically composed of only four elements, earth, air, fire and water, each with its own specific quality: dry, cold, warm and moist respectively.

The concept of qualities had been suggested a little earlier by another early medical authority Alcmaeon (about 500 B.C.), belonging to the same school. He viewed health as the physiological balance between two pairs of opposite qualities: dry-moist and cold-warm. When any one of the qualities occurs in excess, the balance is disturbed; and this is disease. The physician must, in that case, introduce into the system the opposite quality, so that the quality in excess is counter-balanced.

Empedocles improved upon this notion, and taught that the body was constituted of the four elements in varying proportions, and that alterations in the associated qualities were incidental to life. Opposition of qualities determined the state of health or its disturbance. Hippocrates worked on these two basic ideas, (the four elements and the phenomenon of opposition), and propounded his theory of humours.

The four elements with their respective qualities (viz. earth-*dry*, air-*cold*, fire-*warm*, water-*moist*) are responsible for the four humours in the body; blood, yellow-bile, black bile and phlegm. The humours were characterized by combinations of qualities: blood (warm and moist), yellow-bile (warm and dry), black-bile (cold and dry), phlegm (cold and moist).

The four humours occur in individuals in different proportions. This variation is responsible for all the individual differences with regard to physical and mental abilities, dispositions and susceptibility to disease. When the proportion of the humours in their admixture is proper, the condition is known as *eucrasia*, which is reflected in health. When there is an imbalance in the quality of humours in the body, the condition is *dyscrasia*, symptomatic of ailment or disease, a state of stress.

The theory further shows that the condition of *dyscrasia* or stress would automatically be productive of a curative process; to correct the imbalance or restore the equilibrium is a natural urge. There is a constitutional provision and facility for this: the heat of the body. It drains off the excess of the humour that has brought about dyscrasia. The draining off was called 'crisis'; and it was supposed to take several forms such as sweating, purging, blood-letting (haemorrhage). The concept of heat within the body was again a contribution of Empedocles. It is this heat that restores the state of balance (eucrasia).

The dynamics of the four humours is related to natural variations that are seasonal, climatic or elemental. The natural tendency of one of the humours to dominate over the others in a season, and the characteristic ailments that would be manifested thereby are noted. Blood in spring, yellow-bile in summer, black-bile in autumn, and phlegm in winter are on the ascendant.

The theory of humour lost its ground in Greek medicine in course of time. Eristratus of Chios (c. 290 B.C.), whose anatomical knowledge and studies on brain gave a new dimension to ancient medicine, opposed the doctrine of four elements as well as the theory of humours. He looked upon the body as constituted of concrete atoms. Humour, in its original meaning, was a 'fluid' comparable to the Indian idea of *rasa*, and did not have an anatomical location. Asclepiades of Bythria (c. 125 B.C.) also rejected the relevance of the theory of humours to diagnosis or treatment.

The Hippocratic theory was revived by Galen (A.D. 130-200), who incorporated the notion of four humours in his concept of pathology. However, he propounded the idea of a 'spirit' (pneuma) to explain the favourable and unfavourable dynamics of the humours. Theophilus of Protospatharius (A.D. 610-641) was greatly influenced by the views of Galen, and the theory of humours was again popular in the medical world.

When Greek medicine moved, during the Middle Ages, to Constantinople and then to Syria and finally to Arabia, the theory of humours was widely accepted. The medical school at Jundi-Shapur (founded c. A.D. 480) which became celebrated in the Abbasid world during the eighth century, was mostly Greek in its orientation, and regarded Galen as almost an oracle. The physicians who studied here and spread the medical wisdom and practice all over the Middle East accepted the four qualities (cold, warm, dry, moist), the four elements (earth, water, fire, air), and the four humours (blood, yellow-bile, black bile and phlegm).

The old Greek notion that health was a matter of balance between the humours continued to inspire the Arab physicians. But the humours in normalcy also would not be perfectly balanced: qualities and quantities would depend upon several factors such as the age of the individual and season of the year. The bodily organs also had an impact upon the dynamics of humours. Ordinarily, however, they mix evenly, and that is what we call health. Excess of a quality or a humour may vitiate this even mixture; that quality needs to be suppressed, or that humour isolated, in order that normal mixture may be restored. This is what the physician's drugs and treatments seek to achieve.

Of the humours, the two biles are to an extent stored in the bodily organs, the yellow-bile in gall-bladder and black-bile in spleen. The stored portion of the humours do not enter into the admixture of the humours. A humour may become vitiated by combination with another humour in excess, or by a quality that is not natural to it. This is symptomatic of disease.

H

Hārīta: Hārīta was an ancient physician: one of the six disciples of ĀTREYA. A *Saṁhitā* in his name is available (printed, Calcutta 1887). But it does not seem to be an old work. The work is said to have been composed by Hārīta, but the spokesman is Ātreya; hence called ĀTREYA-SAṀHITĀ also [*See* ĀTREYA-SAṀHITĀ].

There are citations in medical works from Hārīta, since lost, and his views are frequently mentioned as authoritative. Thirst, according to him, is the strongest and most irresistible of the urges (tṛshṇā garīyasī ghorā sadyah prāṇavināśinī). One should not sleep immediately after taking food; even a healthy man would fall ill if he does so ('bhuktvā svapnam na seveta, svastho'pyasukhito bhavet).

Many formulae, especially of medicated ghees, are ascribed to him (Hārītokta): Kaṭuka-ghṛta, Mahā-vasādya-ghṛta in haemorrhage (rakta-pitta); Laśuna-ghṛta in jaundice (kāmalā) and inflammation (śosha), and Mahānīla-ghṛta in several ailments, e.g., leucoderma (śvitra), erysipelas (sarpī), abscess (vidradhi), ulcer (vraṇa), insanity (unmāda) and memory disorders (apasmṛti). The last mentioned appears to have been popular (atiprasiddha) during the days of TĪSAṬA.

The printed edition consists of seven divisions (sthānas) and 88 chapters in all. The last division is an appendix (pariśishta), dealing with earlier medical literature. The first division (12 chapters) or (prathama or Annapānaka-Sthāna) is introductory: it treats of food and drink, health, hygiene, physicians, medical education, tastes and seasonal variations.

The second (7 chapters) or (Dvitīya or Arishta-Sthāna) deals with prognostic details of diseases (like dreams, distorted sensations and messengers).

The third (57 chapters) or (Chikitsā-Sthāna) prescribes treatments for various diseases like dysentery (atisāra), abdominal tumours (gulma), indigestion (mandāgni), loss of appetite (arochaka), colic pain (śūla), anaemia (pāṇḍu), epilepsy (apasmāra), piles (arśa), haemorrhage (raktapitta), dropsy (jalodara), leprosy (kushṭa) and insanity (unmāda). There are also accounts of toxicology (vishatantra), paediatrics (bāla-roga), treatment of burns (agnidagdha), troubles in pregnancy and puerperal diseases and bone-setting (bhagna). There is a chapter on virilification (vājīkaraṇa) also.

The fourth division (4 chapters) (Kalpa-Sthāna) deals with drugs (like harītaki, triphalā and rosona) and medicinal preparations. The fifth (6 chapters) (Sūtra-Sthāna) deals with dosage of medicines, weights and measures, medicated oils, treatment methods like rectal injections, clysters, enema and venesection.

The last division (1 chapter only) (Śārīra-Sthāna) deals with anatomical details of the human body, especially in the foetal stage.

Hemādri: He is the author of *Āyurveda-Rasāyana*, an incomplete commentary on *AHr*. Son of KĀMADEVA, he was minister (śrī-karaṇādhipa) to the Yādava king of Devagiri, MAHĀDEVA (1260-71), and his son RĀMACHANDRA-DEVA (1271-1309). His fame rests on the encyclopaedic work, *Chaturvarga-chintāmanı*.

The commentary on *AHr* was composed sometime between 1271 and 1309, for he refers in the prefatory verse to King Rāmachandra deva (Rāmasya rājñah śrīkaraneshvadhi, v.6). He describes himself as a physician (agadaṅkāreṇa Hemādriṇā)

He encouraged many men of letters, among whom was the celebrated VOPADEVA. [*See* ĀYURVEDA-RASĀYANA]

Hikmat-Prakāśa: A treatise on Yunāni (pārasī-pratibiṁba) system of medicine in metrical Sanskrit by MAHĀDEVA, son of BĀLAKṚSHṆA. It is in three parts. The first part deals with physiological constituents, potency, urine examination, etc.; the second part enumerates the drugs with their properties and use; and the third part contains medicinal preparations. The author has himself described this work as 'a curious one' (vichitram). The work was completed in A.D. 1773 (Khemraj Srikrishnadas, Bombay, 1913)

Hiraṇyāksha: An ancient physician (also called Kuśika) whose views on the common origin and disease and on the tastes are quoted by Charaka (*CS*, Sū.sth., chap. 25, yajjah-purushīyam 14 and 15 and chap. 26, Ātreya-Bhadrakāpyīyam), and who is also cited in *VyMk* (in the section on the diseases of children).

He figures among the sages who had assembled to discuss with the venerable Ātreya-Punarvasu about the sources of the human constitution (yaj-jah-purushah), which is a configuration (rāśih) of the soul, sense-organs, sense-objects and mind. The problem was a prelude to determine the origin of diseases. He speaks immediately after VĀRYOVIDA, who propounds that the tastes (rasas) are responsible for the living being as well as the diseases. This view is rejected by HIRAṆYĀKSHA.

He was an adherent of the ancient Sāṁkhya school (esha sāṁkhyair ādyaih parīkshitah), which held that the human constitution is derived from six primary elements (shaḍ-dhātujah purushah, five material elements and consciousness, khādayaś chetanā shashṭha dhātavah purushah, q.Chkp). He concludes that diseases also emerge from the same source, viz., the six elements (rogah shaḍ-dhātujas tathā).

As regards the number of *rasas*, he held that they were four (chatvāro rasāh): sweet and favourable (svādur hitah), sweet but not favourable (svādur ahitah), not sweet but favourable (asvādur hitah), neither sweet nor favourable (asvādur ahitah). Sweet is explained by *Chkp* as 'desirable' *(abhīṣṭam)* and favourable as 'unharmful' *(āyatāvanapakārī) (CS,* Sū.sth., 26)

This discussion takes place in another conference of sages Bhadrakāpya, Śakunta, Maudgalya, Hiraṇyāksha (Kuśika) and others with Ātreya in the delightful garden, Chaitra-ratha. All the sages who participated in this discussion are described as learned and aged (śruta-vayo-vṛddhā) and great sages known for their self-restraint (jitātmāno maharshyah) (*CS*, I, i, 3-6).

Hṛdaya-dīpikā: A glossary of drugs giving only synonyms prepared by VOPADEVA, son of the physician KEŚAVA (author of *Siddha-mantra*) and pupil of DHANEŚVARA. It is little more than a list of synonyms, and follows the style of PARYĀYA-RATNA-MĀLĀ. The work is in 8 sections, and the last section ('miscellaneous', *miśrakavarga*) includes details other than drugs (like diet and five-fold treatment). The drugs mentioned here are taken directly from *AH*r; hence the title of the work.

The author was a court-physician to Mahādeva, the Yādava ruler of Devagiri (A.D. 1260-71), and was patronized by the celebrated Hemādri, the King's minister and adviser, who also wrote a commentary on *AHr* (*Āyurveda-rasāyana*). Vopadeva has written several other works including a gloss on his father's *Siddha-mantra* (Prakāśa) and a commentary on *Śārṅgadhara-saṁhitā* (*Gūḍhārtha-dīpikā*).

I

Indra: A celebrated and colourful hero in *RV*, Indra learnt medicine from the Aśvins and taught the sages Bhāradvāja and Dhanvantari, who crystallized the Indian therapeutics and surgery. He is son of Kaśyapa and is always pictured as a youth (kumāraka); he is also regarded as the youngest of gods (kanīna, 'the little one'). He is extolled as the offspring of the Sky and Earth; and numerous hymns of *RV* record his heroic deeds, the most illustrious of which was the slaying of the dragon, Vṛtra.

He is associated with the invigorating drink, soma, which has been praised in as many as 120 hymns in *RV*, including an entire 'maṇḍala' (the 9th). He is said to have derived his strength, courage and goodwill from this drink (*RV*, 1,61,7; 3,36,3; 4,10,5 etc), which was recovered for him by his associate Vishṇu (*RV*, 3,48,4). The excellent qualities of this 'herbal preparation' have been listed in the *RV*: it tones up the body, eliminates the ailments, nourishes the limbs, cheers up and exhilarates; it is an antedote to depression and melancholy, and is said to stir up good and pleasant thoughts.

His knowledge of medicine is extolled in *RV* (2,23,7), and his association with the Aśvins, the divine physicians, is celebrated in sautrāmani-ritual. He is claimed to have restored eyesight to Parāvṛja and to have helped Śroṇa to recover the ability to walk (2,15,7). He is recorded to have cured Apālā of her skin-disease (8,91,7). His skill as a surgeon has also been mentioned (8,1,12; *AV* 14,2,47), as also his knowledge of snakes and scorpions (10,4,14).

AV adds that Indra was an expert in healing mental illnesses (6,111,4) and that he gave many recipes (5,25,4-6). He was also responsible for many a germicide (3,37,8; 5,23,1). Foetus was 'protected' by him (5,25, 4-6). His name is mentioned in connection with the disease āsrāva (2,3,6). *Vājasaneyi-saṁhitā* (35,46) addresses a prayer to Indra for health and medicines.

A tonic to prolong life (rasāyana) is ascribed to him. Known as Aindrī-rasāyana, it is said to have been taught by him to Bhṛgu, Atri and other sages. Hārītakī-lehya is also associated with his name.

Indu: Indu or Indu-kara is the author of *Śaśilekhā,* the only commentary on *Ashṭāṅga-Saṁgraha* that is extant. It is probably a South Indian work.

His date is uncertain. But as HEMĀDRI quotes him, he is earlier than A.D. 1260. [*See* ŚAŚILEKHĀ]

Indu-Nighaṇṭu: Cited as an authority by *Kshīra-svāmin* (11th century commentary on *Amara-kosha*) and the author of *Siva-kosha*, this must have been a pharmacological glossary of considerable popularity. The author of this work, Indu, does not appear to be the same as the commentator on *AHr*. The work, however, is no longer extant.

J

Jaijjaṭa: Jaijjata, also known as Jejjaṭa, Jaiyyaṭa is the author of the earliest commentary on *SS* (around 5th century), quoted by Ḍalhaṇa.

He is said to have been a student of VĀGBHAṬA. The name suggests that he was from Kāshmīr. [*See* SUŚRUTA-SAṀHITĀ]

Jalpa-kalpa-taru: This is a philosophical gloss on *CS*, by GAṄGĀDHARA-KAVIRĀJ (VS 1856-1942), a renowned Ayurvedic physician of modern times who was also the leader of renaissance in Indian medicine.

Jīvaka: A renowned physician during the days of the Buddha, Jīvaka was a specialist in paediatrics (kaumāra-bhṛtya), one of the eight aspects of Indian medicine.

According to the Buddhist text, *Mahāvagga*, the Tibetan accounts preserved in Kah-gyur, and the account in Buddhagosha's Pāli commentary *Sumaṅgalavilāsinī* on the canonical *Dīgha-Nikāya,* he was a physician to the Buddha himself and the king Biṁbisāra. Son of Sālavatī, a courtezan of Vesāli, and the prince Abhaya, grandson of Biṁbisāra, he was inspired to become a physician when, as an youngster, he saw a physician who received his fees only when the patient was cured and not otherwise. He learnt some medicine in his home-town, but went to Takshaśilā to specialize in surgery (including "the art of skull-opening") and learnt for seven years under the renowned master there, Ātreya by name (not the Ātreya who taught Agnivesá and others). He held the view that one should not learn medicine at all if one was not interested in learning it thoroughly.

Many remarkable cures are ascribed to him; and his treatment as contained in the legends included a quick cure for jaundice, laparotomy, cranial operations and easy delivery. His fame, however, rests as a child specialist.

Bower Mss. contains a formula of his for diseases of children (2, p.176): "Clerodendron siphonanthus (bhargi), long pepper (pippali), Stephania hermandi folia (patha), gynoandropsis pentaphylla (payasa), with honey (madhunā saha), this linctus (lihet) would cure emesis (chardi) that is due to the deranged śleshma."

Chakradattam contains another recipe (Saureśvara-ghṛita) who is said to cure elephantiasis (ślīpada), sprue (grahaṇī) and oedema (śvayathu). It is also said to be a cardiac tonic (hṛdya) and anthelminite (koshṭha-krimi-vināśanam). Yet another recipe is said to be especially good for children (kumārāṇām sukhāvaham), a powder of (drākshā), fagonia arabica (durālabha).

K

Kalyāṇa-kāraka: This is a comprehensive medical treatise in lucid Sanskrit verse, written by the Jaina ascetic UGRĀDITYA (about A.D. 850) on mount Rāma-giri in Āndhra Pradesh. It deals with all the branches of medicine in two parts and 25 chapters. (Ed. by Vardhmāna Pārśvanātha Śāstri, Sakhārām Nemichandra Series No. 129, Sholāpur, 1940).

The author claims to have consulted numerous earlier medical texts by Jaina authors, such as on 'minor surgery' by PŪJYAPĀDA, on surgery (śalya-tantra) by PĀTRASVĀMIN, on toxicology and pacification of the evil dispositions of planets (vishogra-graha-śamana-vidhi) by SIDDHA-SENA; on paediatrics (chikitsā..śiśūnām) by DAŚARATHA and MEGHANĀDA, and on rejuvenation (vaidyam vṛshyam) by SIṀHA-NĀDA (20, 85). These, however, are no longer available, or they may be in manuscripts unnoticed.

The work assumes a typical Jaina outlook in rejecting the use of animal food and alcohol while treating diseases, and assumes a position against even Charaka in this regard. Diseases (āmaya) and meat (māṁsa) are both alike caused by sin (pāpajatvāt), by the three doshas, and by the involvement of bodily constituents (mala-dhātu-nibandhanāt); and, therefore, meat cannot be employed to cure a disease (na pratīkārakam). It is wrong to argue that plants and meat are not different, on the ground that both are living beings. Meat is living substance (jīva-śarīra), but all living substances are not meat: neem is a tree, but not all trees are neem! The work recommends only the medicines derived from the vegetable kingdom, and that too in little quantity (*svalpam*) and taken in an agreeable manner (*sukham pathyatamam*).

The enumeration and description of diseases here follow a line that is rather unique, and quite different from the scheme usually followed (as eg. in *MN*). The major diseases are classified neatly in three categories according to disturbances of the three *doshas*. Most of the ailments listed in works like *MN* are here classed as minor (kshudra-roga). The work gives an account of the methods of rejuvenation also. Mercury has been mentioned but barely and briefly. Treatment procedures like cautery, enemata and surgery have also been indicated.

The involvement of occult methods and astrology in medicine can already be seen in this work; but only as diagnostic aids. Inquiry (praśna), oracular utterances (āgama), omens (śakuna), supernatural indications (nimitta), dreams (svapna), prophesies (divya-kathita) and consideration of stellar positions (lagna) are said to help the physician to understand the life-span (viz., curability or otherwise) of the patient.

It is curious that the expression 'Vaidya' (for medicine, treatment or physician) has here been derived from 'vidyā' (the perfect and omniscient vision); the physician (vaidya) is said to be one who is proficient in the science that has emerged from vidyā (I, 18).

This work was translated into Kannada by the poet JAGADDALA-SOMANĀTHA in A.D. 1150. But this poet appears to regard the author of the original work as Pūjyapāda. [*See* UGRĀDITYA].

Kaṅkāyana: This ancient physician who belonged to the Bāhlīka region (Bāhlīka-bhishak) has been quoted by Charaka (*CS*, Sū. sth., ch.25, *yajjah-purushīya*, 22 and 23; ch.26, *Atreya-Bhadrakāpyīyam*, 8; and Śā. sth., ch.6, *śarīra-vichayam*, 21).

He appears as a participant in the conference on the origin of diseases (I, 25), opposing the argument of Bhāradvāja that diseases are natural emergences during the course of evolution, (bhava-hetuh svabhāvas tu vyādhīnām), as natural as the emergence of the five material elements. Kaṅkāyana disapproves of the idea of naturalness of diseases on the ground that human effort in the case would be unwarranted and futile (na hi ārambha-phalam bhavet). He holds that it is the creator with infinite intentions (srashṭā tu amita-saṁkalpah) that is responsible for the happiness and unhappiness in the world and for man (chetanāchetanasya asya jagatah sukha-dukhayoh).

He appears again in the discussion in the Chaitra-ratha garden on the number of tastes (*rasas*) in the presence of Ātreya (1, 26). He argues that tastes are really infinite (aparisamkhyeyā rasā), and that they are apprehended only on the basis of innumerable factors like location, quality, action and individual differences (āśraya-guṇa-karma-samsvāda-visheshāṇām aparisamkhyeyatyāt; *Chkp* explains 'samsvāda' as svasamvedya, viz. individual difference in apprehension).

The third place in *CS* where he appears is in connection with the discussion on foetal development (IV, 6). He holds that 'heart' (hṛdayam) is the first organ to be developed, because it is there that consciousness is located (chetanādhishṭhānatvāt).

Kāśyapa: He is an early medical authority cited by CHARAKA and is probably the son of MARĪCHI. According to him, the chief source of human ailments is the aberration in the Śleshman (*CS*, Sū. Sth., 12, 12). He is also mentioned in the *Bower Mss*, where his prescriptions for some diseases of children (like diarrhoea, vomiting, hiccough, cough, retention of discharges, morbid secretion of urine, gripes, worms, jaundice, diphtheria and skin troubles) are given (vv. 1010-1040, pp. 170-172). A morbid change in the child's appearance is here ascribed to an attack by a demoness (Pūtanā), but is sought to be remedied by a pill!

He is cited in *AHr*, and discussed in *NiS*. The view ascribed to him is that in the third month of foetal growth, all the sense-organs and parts of the body get formed simultaneously (yugapat).

He is sometimes identified with Jīvaka (not the famous contemporary of the Buddha, but an earlier physician, hence designated Vrddha-Jīvaka). But the work in his name makes him a teacher of a young man Jīvaka who was turned into a venerable old man to give greater credibility.

A *saṁhitā* is available in his name (*See* KĀŚYAPA-SAṀHITA). There are references to a tantra in his name, but it is not extant. There is another work called *Kāśyapīya-roga-nidānam*, attributed to him; but it is a recent work. Several formulae are ascribed to him (e.g., Traiphala-ghṛtam, Kāśyapīyaguḍikā).

Kāśyapa-saṁhitā: Written in simple Sanskrit ascribed to Kāśyapa, this work closely resembles *CS* in style, divisions and approach. It belongs to an early strata of medical literature in India. A Ms. of this work was recovered from the Nepāl Durbār Library, Khaṭmaṇḍu and edited by Yādav Trikam Āchārya (Publ. by Hemarāj Paṇḍit, NS, Bombay) in 1938.

The work is in eight divisions (names of which are similar to those of *CS*, except the last one, here called khila), and 200 chapters (the last division, supplementary containing 80). The work is now available in a mutilated state with many sections missing. The work traces the transmission of medical knowledge, as in *CS*, from Brahmā through Daksha, the Aśvins and Indra. From Indra, however, the account here directly proceeds to Kāśyapa and three other sages: Vaśishṭha, Atri and Bhṛgu.

Kāśyapa is said to have passed it on to a youngster, Jīvaka (son of Sage Ṛchīka), who wrote a medical tract based on Kāśyapa's teachings. Because of the author's youth, the sages did not take the work seriously. But when, by a miracle, the youth was transformed into a grand old man (Vṛddha-Jīvaka), his work became celebrated and popular. It came to be known as *Vṛddha-Jīvaka-tantra.*

The work was lost in course of time, but a spirit, Anāyāsa by name, had preserved it out of compassion for the suffering folk (loka-bhūtaye). A descendant of Jīvaka, Vātsya by name, recovered the text from the spirit, redacted and abridged it (sañchikshepa), and made it once more popular. He also added the supplementary section (Khila-Sthāna) to the "eight" divisions of the original work. (The available work has eight Sthānas, including the Khila-Sthāna; the missing Sthāna is Nidāna-Sthāna.)

The exponent here Marīchi-Kāśyapa, who is mentioned in *CS* (*Sū. Sth.* 1, 12 and *Śā. Sth.* 6, 21), and the pupil is Bhārgava. The work opens with "Thus says the revered Kāśyapa" (iti ha smāha bhagavān Kāśyapah). According to the work, Āyurveda as revealed by Indra to the four sages (Kāśyapa and others) is the source and support of the four Vedas (āyurvedam āśrayante vedāh), like the four fingers of the hand depending upon the thumb. The four Vedas teach the three-fold values of life (trivarga: dharma, artha and kāma); Āyurveda deals with the source of these values, the health of the individual.

The philosophical foundation of the medical system expounded here is Sāṁkhya, and the general approach is to obtain knowledge concerning cause, symptoms and treatment (hetu-liṅga-aushadha-jñāna) of diseases, as in *CS*. The work mainly deals with midwifery, gynaecology and diseases of children. It is said here that of the eight divisions of Āyurveda, paediatrics (kaumārabhṛtya) is the best. Rickets (phakka) is dealt with in some detail, and is explained as caused by drinking the mother's milk which is vitiated by kapha. A medicated oil, Kaṭutaila, is prescribed for disorders of spleen.

The welfare of the newborn child is said to be secured by worshipping Shąshṭī (the six-faced divinity of the sixth day of the lunar month, presiding over the health of infants). There is also a mention of the Buddhist Mātaṅgī-Vidyā, and employment of the typical Jaina expressions utsarpiṇī and avasarpiṇī to denote the ascending and descending phases of the time-cycle. Many formulae included in the *Bower Mss.* are from Kāśyapa.

Another work under the same title is available in the Tanjore Library (No.10780), but it does not appear to be an ancient one. It deals with several diseases like fever, dysentery, piles and nervous ailments. It is in the form of a dialogue between Pārvatī (who questions) and Parameśvara (who answers) on mount Kailāsa. The initial questions concern sins, diseases and hells. But the introductory portion mentions that some Gautama asked questions concerning medicine of the great sage Kāśyapa, who is described as "brilliant like the Sun." The work, in addition to normal medicines, prescribes also magic and religious rituals as curative methods.

Khotanese medical text: A bilingual manuscript in 70 folios (11¾×31″) written in mixed Sanskrit and Khotanese discovered in Eastern Turkistan and now preserved in the India Office Library (CH 11003), this text contains medical prescriptions in metrical form (cf. H.W. Bailey, *Codices Khotaneses*, Copenhagen, 1938; Sten Konow, *A Medical Text in Khotanese*, Eng. Transl., 1940).

This is principally a work on Toxicology (agada), although it also contains cures for many common ailments like fever, cough, hiccough, eye-diseases, troubled respiration and consumption. The text not only specifies drugs (e.g., aśvagandha for cough, respiratory disorders, consumption etc.; Kalyāṇaka for hiccough, insomnia, fever, piles, insanity etc.; bālagarbha for insomnia, impurity of blood, consumption, scurvy, etc.) but describes methods of preparing medicines. More than 90 preparations are included here, along with names of diseases.

The authorship of the work is unknown, but the narrative is addressed to some Jīvaka (probably the famous physician, contemporary of the Buddha). The invocatory verses mentions Brahma, the first exponent of the science of medicine, and the sages who were treasures of adept wisdom (siddha-vidyā-rishis) in India (Jaṁbudvīpa). Later the name of the great Atreya is also mentioned.

The use of incantations (mantras) is recommended both while preparing the drugs and when administering them, especially in cases of diseases due to poisoning (agada) and evil influences. Medicines are sought to be consecrated or invigorated by the employment of sacred formulae.

Kshārapāṇi: One of the early masters of medicine, he was a contemporary and fellow-student of AGNIVEŚA, who provided the basic text for *Charaka-Saṁhitā*. A student of Ātreya, he wrote his own medical treatise, which unfortunately was lost in course of time. But his views have been cited in several later works such as *VyK* (Śrīkaṇṭha-datta) and *Tattva-Chandrikā* (Śivadāsa-Sena). One of his views is that, although sleep during daytime is unhealthy, one who loses sleep during night for any reason will benefit by sleep during daytime for half the time lost in the night (cited in *VyK*).

Some formulae are ascribed to him, such as Bilvādya-ghṛta for diseases of the spleen (plīha) and Nīla-ghṛta for leucoderma (śvitra).

Kumāra-śira: Called Kumāra-śira-Bharadvāja, he is quoted by Charaka as an ancient physician, contemporaneous with ĀTREYA (*CS*, Sū. sth., ch.25, 20-21; ch. 26-8; and Śā. sth., ch. 6, 21).

As one of the participants in the conference on the origin of diseases, he argued that diseases are naturally caused (bhavahetuh svabhāvas tu vyādhīnāṃ), even as solidity, liquid, warmth and combustion are natural emergences of the five elements (earth, water, air and fire). (1, 25, 20 and 21).

In the discussion on the number of tastes (1, 26, 8), he supports the view that tastes are five in number (pañcha-rasāh), and he relates them to the five elements: earth, water, fire, air and ether (bhaumodakāgneya-vāyavyāntarikshāh).

As regards the problem of foetal development (IV, 6), he argues that head (śirah) is the first organ to get formed, for that is the locus for all sense-organs (sarvendriyāṇām adhishṭhānam iti).

L

Lāḍyāyana: An ancient specialist in toxicology, he is also celebrated for his classification of insects and reptiles (kīṭa) according to their dottings (kaṭu), markings (lekhā), wings (paksha), mouth with antennae or nipper (mukha), claws (nakha), filaments or sharp hairs (saṁślishṭa-paksha-roma), humming (svana), size (pramāṇa), bodily structure (saṁsthāna), sexual organs (liṅga), poisons (visha) and the poisonous effect (vīrya). He is quoted by ḌALHAṆA in his commentary on *SS*, Kalp. Sth., 8.

Lolimba-rāja (or Lolaṁba-rāja): He is the author of a curious medical work in the form of a poem with all the usual literary embellishments, *Vaidya-jīvana*.

Son of Divākara-bhaṭṭa, he was a resident of Junnār in Puṇe dist. (Mahārāshṭra). He had married a Muslim girl, and after her death, turned an ascetic. He was a devotee of Durgā. He had the title 'the prince of poets' (Kavi-bādshāh).

The Ms. of his *Vaidya-Jīvana* dated A.D. 1608 has been found, and so he must have lived before 1600.

Two other works from his pen, *Vaidyāvtaaṁsa* and *Chamatkāra-chintāmaṇi* deal with medical subjects.

He was also a Marāṭhī poet. [*See* VAIDYA-JĪVANA].

M

Madana-pāla-nighaṇṭu: This is a popular medical glossary compiled by MADANA-PĀLA, the scion of the Gahaḍvāra family which ruled over Kanauj between A.D. 1098 and 1109 according to Rājendralāl Mitra. Bhāṇḍārkar would assign this work to *circa* A.D. 1375 but Narahari, the author of *Rāja-nighaṇṭu* (between A.D.1235 and 1250) has consulted this work.

It is extensive in bulk and deals with a large number of drugs (dravyas). Medicinal qualities of as many as 870 plants have been given. However, the author claims that his work is neither too brief nor too voluminous (nāti-laghur na chāti vipulah). The last section, entitled 'miscellaneous' (miśraka), contains useful information about healthful daily conduct (dina-charyā) and in different seasons (ṛtu-charyā).

The work is also called *Madana-vinoda* (Banaras, 1875). It is in 14 sections, containing 2,250 verses. [*See* NIGHAṆṬU].

Madana-vinoda: Also called Madana-pāla-nighaṇṭu, it is designed to be a pharmacological glossary, "not too brief, nor too prolix, containing names of drugs that are well known, and giving the details of properties etc. of those drugs." The work in 13 chapters (abhayā, etc., śunthī, etc., camphor, etc., gold, etc., *vaṭa,* etc., grapes, etc., and vegetables, drinks, sweets, cereals, preparations of food, meat and miscellaneous) was completed in A.D. 1374 (samvat 1431).

Among metals zinc (yaśada) has not been mentioned. But among the drugs introduced by outside influences are mentioned opium (ahiphena, Papever somniferum), bhaṅg, Pārasika-yavāni (Hyseyamus niger), mārjārī, sindhūrī (Bixa orellama), Sulaimānī, Kharjūr (Anacardium occidentale), Kharbūj (cucumis melo), badām (Prunus amygdalus), aṅjūra (Ficus carica), guñjan, etc.

The author, MADANA-PĀLA, was the son of Sādhāraṇa, a scion of the Ṭāka dynasty of the town Kāshṭhā. He was a nobleman, who patronized many literary men, including VIŚVEŚVARA (the author of *Madana-pārijāta)* and RAMARĀJA (the author of *Rasa-ratna-dīpa*).

This work has been very popular with the physicians, especially in the northern regions of the country. (Naval Kisor Press, Lucknow, 1917; ed. Nandakisor Sastri, Varanasi, 1933; Gangavishnu Sri Krishnadas, Bombay 1954).

Mādhava-dravya-guṇa: A work of pharmacological interest, it seeks to summarize the "bhāva-svabhāva-vāda of antiquity" (intro. verse). What this doctrine was, however, cannot be ascertained from the contents of this voluminous work of about 900 verses.

The concluding verse claims that the author has gathered therein all relevant matter from the works of Suśruta, Charaka, Parāśara, Bhattāra-Hari-Chandra, Bheḍa, Vaideha, Hārīta and others.

The work appears to follow closely *Soḍhala-nighantu (see* under S) probably of 12th century; and it has been relied upon heavily by Toḍarānanda's classic of the 16th century. It has been cited by Vopadeva (13th century), Āḍhamalla (14th century), Śivadāsa-sena (15th century) and in *Śiva-kosha* (17th century).

The authorship of the work is uncertain. He is said to be the grandson of the celebrated Śrīkaṇṭha-datta (disciple of Vijaya-rakshita) and father of Purushottama, another pharmacological writer.

Mādhava-kara: Author of the celebrated work on pathology, *Rug-viniśchaya* (more popularly known as *Mādhava-Nidāna*) and also of a glossary of medical terms known as *Ratna-mālā* (or *Paryāya-ratna-mālā*, ed. by Tārāpada Chaudhury, Patnā Univ.).

He was the son of INDU-KARA and a native of Śilāhrada in Bengal (as mentioned in his *Ratna-mālā*). The suffix 'kara' in his name suggests that he belonged to a Bengali family (according to Gananath Sen). He is sometimes but wrongly identified with Mādhava, the brother of the famous Sāyaṇa.

He is assigned to seventh century, because he is quoted by VṚNDA in the eighth century and his work was translated into Persian during the reign of the Kaliph Harun-al-Rashid (*c.* A.D. 786), on the testimony of al-Beruni.

Other works ascribed to him are *Āyurveda-prakāśa* and *Rasa-Śāstra* (or *Rasa-kaumudī*) [*See* MĀDHAVA-NIDĀNA].

Mādhava-nidāna: A popular and comprehensive work on pathology (nidāna), it has been an indispensable aid to physicians for over a thousand years. There is a saying that this work is supreme in the field of pathology (nidāne Mādhavah śreshṭhah). So named after the author, the real title of the work is *Roga-viniśchaya* (or *Rug-viniśchaya*), the first work on pathology.

The work is an elaborate consideration of causes, symptoms, complications and treatments in 73 sections. The first section deals with the five factors necessary for proper diagnosis of a disease: nidāna (cause), pūrva-rūpa (premonitory symptoms), rūpa (manifested symptoms), *upaśaya* ('applied therapeutics', to trace the cause from the effect), and saṁprāpti (development of disease).

The rest of the work deals with diseases: fever (jvara), dysentery (atisāra), chronic diarrhoea (grahaṇī), piles (arśa), dyspepsia (agni-māndya), anaemia (pāṇḍu), jaundice (kāmalā), chlorosis (halīmaka), haemorrhage (rakta-pitta), pulmonary tuberculosis (rāja-yakshma), cough (kāsa), hiccough (hikkā), asthma (śvāsa), hoarseness (svara-bheda), loss of appetite (arochaka), vomiting (chardi), abnormal thirst (tṛshṇā), fainting (mūrchchhā), giddiness (bhrama), apoplexy (saṁnyāsa), alcoholism (madātyaya), insanity (unmāda), epilepsy (apasmāra), convulsions (ākshepaka), tetanus (dhanurvāta), hemiplegia (pakshāghāta), facial paralysis (ardita), paraplegia (ūrustaṁbha), gout (vāta-rakta), delirium (ati-pralāpa), rheumatism (āma-vāta), colic (śūla), gastralgokenosis (pariṇāma-śūlā), acidity (amla-pitta), constipation (ānāha), abdominal tumour (gulma), diseases of the heart (hṛd-roga), stranguary (mūtra-kṛchchha), obstructed micturition (mūtrāghāta), calculus (aśmarī), urinary diseases (prameha), diabetes (udaka-meha), other associated ailments, obesity (medo-vṛddhi), splenic enlargement (plīhodara), ascites (jalodara), intestinal obstruction (baddha-gudodara), dropsy (śotha), enlargements (vṛddhi), goitre (gala-gaṇḍa), scrofula (gāṇḍa-mālā), tumours (arbuda), cancer (raktārbuda), elephantiasis (ślīpada), abscess (vidradhi), inflammation (vraṇa-śotha), idiopathic ulcer (śārīra-vraṇa), traumatic wound (sadyo-vraṇa), fracture (asthi-bhaṅga), fistula-in- ano (bhagandara), skin diseases (kushṭha), leprosy (mahā-kushṭha), erysipelas (visarpa), exanthymeta (śīta-pitta), small-pox (masūrikā), minor ailments (kshudra-roga), measles (romantika), diseases of the face, ears, nose and eyes, diseases of the head, diseases of women, diseases of children, and poisons.

The last section gives a list of diseases dealt with. The book ends with a prayer that all living beings be freed from the entire host of ailments (muñchantu jantavas tena nityam ātaṅka-santatim, verse II).

It can be seen that the work draws heavily from *CS* and *SS*. It devotes an entire chapter (66) to small-pox (*masūrikā),* which during the days of *SS* was but a minor ailment.

The work was translated into Arabic under orders from the Kaliphs of Baghdad during the 9th century, and into Italian by Mario Vallduri in 1913-14. Among the editions, Jībānanda Vidyāsāgar's (Calcutta 1876), U.C. Datta's (Calcutta 1880), and Raghunāthprasād-Sītārām's (Bombay 1884) are the earliest ones.

There are many commentaries on it, the most popular among which is *Madhu-kośa* (jointly prepared by VIJAYA-RAKSHITA till 32nd chapter and ŚRĪKAṆṬHA-DATTA (ed. Jībānanda-Vidyāsāgar 1876). Other commentaries include *Ātaṅka-darpaṇa* (by VAIDYA-VĀCHASPATI), *Siddhānta-chandrikā* (by NARASIṂHA), *Subodhinī* (by MADHURA-KĀYASTHA), *Nidāna-pradīpa* and *Nidāna-ṭippaṇī*.

Madhu-kosha: Also known as (*Vyākhyā - Madhu-Kosha)* this is a commentary on *Madhava Nidana* by VIJAYA-RAKSHITA (sections 1 to 32) and his student ŚRĪKAṆṬHA-DATTA (section 33 till the end). The date of this excellent commentary is 13th century. The earliest available Ms. is dated A.D. 1529.

The commentary explains the actual title of *MN*, viz., Roga-Viniśchaya as the specific (viśesheṇa) determination of the nature and course of disease in terms of its aetiology (vātajatvādi) and prognosis (sādhyāsādhyatvādirūpena).

The commentary quotes *CS, SS* and *AHr* extensively. It also refers to the views of Jaijjaṭa, Vāpya-Chandra (frequently), Kīrti-Kuṇḍa (Kārtika), Sudānta-Sena, Bhaṭṭāra-Harichandra, Gadādhara, Pālakāpya, Karavīra, Parāśara, Hārīta, Bhoja, Jatūkarṇa, Gayasena, Chakra, Bhāluki, Kharanāda, and Dṛḍhabala. It distinguishes between Vṛddha-Suśruta ('elder Suśruta', the original compiler of the teachings of Dhanvantari) and Suśruta (the author of the present *SS*). The 'Kāshmīrī Recension' (Kāśmīra-pāṭha) of *CS* has been mentioned.

A *Bhāluki-tantra* is often quoted; we are not sure if this is the same as the *Bhela-Saṁhitā* that has come down to us.

The commentary becomes especially important, for many of the medical works from which it quotes are now lost, and the citations are often full verses.

Among the early editions of this commentary, Jībānanda-Vidyāsāgar's (1876) and the Nirṇaya-sāgar edition (along with another commentary Ātaṅka-darpaṇa) may be mentioned. [*See* VIJAYA-RAKSHITA and ŚRĪKAṆṬHA-DATTA].

Marīchi: He is a medical authority cited by Charaka. According to him, diseases are solely caused by the bodily fire (agni) inherent in the metabolic processes (pittāntargata) (*CS, Sū. Sth.,* 12, 11). Probably he held that among the three *doṣhās, pitta* was the dominant. He was also aware of the five-fold division of the functions of pitta: *pāchaka*, *ālochaka*, etc. (*cf.* commentary of Chkp.

on above). Regarding the problem of what organ of the foetus gets initially formed, he held that it was impossible to determine (*CS* Śā. Sth., 6, 21). Charaka mentions in this context that he belonged to Kāśyapa clan (Marīchih Kāśyapah). But in the *Kāśyapa-Saṁhitā* that is available, all sense-organs and parts of the body in the foetus are said to get formed simultaneously (yugapat) in the third month (p. 46). The same view is held by Suśruta.

N

Nāgārjuna: He is a redactor (prati-saṁskartā) of *SS* (according to Ḍalhaṇa) and reputed to be the author of the final portion of *SS*, viz., uttara-tantra (according to Cordier). He is author of *Rasaratnākara* and several recipes and formulae.

By all accounts, the most remarkable among Indian thinkers, Nāgārjuna has also been the most enigmatic figure in Indian history. So numerous are the works ascribed to him, and so varied are the accomplishments credited to him, that Western scholars are either inclined to suspect his historicity altogether (e.g., Wissiljew who regarded him as wholly mythical) or assume the existence of several Nāgārjunas (e.g., M. Winternitz who postulated four Nāgārjunas: the Buddhist writer, the Tāntrik writer, the Medical writer and the alchemist).

However, the Indian view (as also the Chinese and Tibetan) has all along held that there was only one Nāgārjuna, who was all these (poet, philosopher, physician, alchemist and saint), although there are many works spuriously attributed to him. He was born a Brahmin but turned a Buddhist, and was intimately associated with the emergence of Mahāyāna branch of Buddhism. He was a native of Vidarbha (modern Berar) in Mahākoshala, but lived for the most part of his life in the monastery on mount Śrī-parvata or Śrī-śaila near Krishṇā river (in Āndhra Pradesh). He was a disciple of the siddha, SARAHA-PĀDA. He was connected with the Nālandā University, and was the teacher of Ārya-deva who later became the chief paṇḍita of that university.

An account of the life and career of Nāgārjuna which was in Sanskrit (and now lost) was translated into Chinese by Kumārajīva in A.D. 401. There are also Tibetan accounts including an elaborate one by the historian Lama Tārānātha. According to these accounts, he succeeded the patriarch Pārśva and administered the Buddhist community for 62 years. He was a friend and counsellor to the Śātavāhana (Hiuen Tsang's So-to-po-ho) king, Gautamī-putra (or Yajña-śrī) Śātakarṇi, who built a monastery for him on Śrī-śaila.

His probable date is hotly debated and is variously given: Fleet, around 57 B.C.; Lassen, around A.D. 23; Vincent Smith, about A.D. 120; S. Beal, A.D. 166-200; Bhaṇḍārkar, about A.D. 278. But since he was a contemporary of Kanishka and the Śātavāhana king according to most accounts (Kumārajīva, Hiuen Tsang, Lāma Tārānātha, and Kalhaṇa's *Rājataraṅgiṇī,* 1, 172 and 173), he may safely be assigned to a period between A.D. 80 and 104.

He was a prolific writer, and wrote on many subjects (philosophy, religion, medicine, chemistry, alchemy); and whatever he wrote became a classic. Among his philosophical writings, *Mūlamādhyamaka-kārikā, Yukti-shashṭhikā, Śūnyatā-saptati, Daśa-bhūmikā-śāstra* and *Māhāyana-viṁśaka* are well known and frequently studied. His *Prajñā-pāramita-sūtra-śastra* (gloss on *Pañchaviṁśati-prajñā-pāramitā*) is a mystical work which made a deep impact on the development of the Mahāyāna sect. His *Suhṛllekha* (letter to his royal friend Śātavāhana, translated into Chinese by Guṇavarma between A.D. 424 and 431) was a short manual that was popularly read and memorized when the Chinese traveller I-Tsing visited the country (7th century).

In the field of medicine, he is reputed to have redacted the whole of *SS*, which probably was in a poor state of preservation during his days. The present shape of *SS* is probably due entirely to Nāgārjuna's reconstruction. The famous commentary on *SS*, Ḍalhaṇa testifies to this fact (*NiS* Sū, sth., 1, 1, yatra yatra paroksho niyogah, tatra tatraiva pratisaṁskartṛ sūtram jñātavyam iti; pratisaṁskartā pī'ha Nāgārjuna eva).

It is also suggested that the last section in *SS* (Uttara-tantra) which was not in the original *SS*, was supplemented by Nāgārjuna (Cordier). It deals with diseases of the eye, ear, nose and head (26 chapters, śālākya), management of the diseases of children (12 chapters, kaumara-bhṛtya), general therapeutics (21 chapters, kāya-chikitsā), insanity and epilepsy (three chapters, bhūta-vidyā) and general considerations such as taste, hygiene, medical terminology and the theory of *doshas* four chapters).

Two other medical works, *ārogya-mañjarī* and *Yoga-sāra* are ascribed to him. the latter has been quoted by VAṄGA-SENA.

The most important contribution of Nāgārjuna, however, is in the application of chemistry, metallurgy and alchemy to medicine. Several works in this field are ascribed to him; e.g. *Rasa-ratnākara* or *Rasendra-maṅgala* (on the use and preparation of mineral drugs), *Rasa-kachchha-puṭa* (on purification of mercury and preparation of mercurial powders, etc.), and *Yoga-śataka* (a book of a hundred recipes also translated into Tibetan; sometimes ascribed to Vararuchi). But the authorship of these works has been a matter of some dispute among scholars.

He is said to have written two works on alchemy, *Lauha-śāstra* (according to *CS*) and *Rasendra-chintāmaṇi* which have not come down to us. There is a *Kaksha-puṭa-tantra* (or *Siddha-chāmuṇḍā),* a work of 1800 verses, in his name; but it is a recent work dealing with magic and witchcraft. *Rati-śāstra* which is in the form of a dialogue between Nāgārjuna and Tuṇḍi on the subject of sex and love, has been ascribed to Nāgārjuna though altogether unjustifiably.

The formulae and recipes that are current in his name include a varti (against cataract), Abhra-rasāyana (for cough, fever, asthma and tuberculosis), Haridrā-khaṇḍa (germicide, remedy for skin ailments, ulcers, fistula, jaundice, etc.), Ghoḍa-choli-rasa (for colic, consumption, intractable cough and asthma), Nāgārjunābhra (for heart-diseases, weakness and indigestion), Rasābhravaṭī, Mṛta-saṁjīvinī-guṭikā, Siddha-rasendra and Nāgārjuna-yoga [*See SS,* RASARATNĀKARA, Nāgārjuna's recipes, and RASA SCHOOL OF MEDICINE].

Nakula: He is the author of a book on the treatment of horses, *Aśva-chikitsā*. Traditionally he is identified with one of the Pāṇḍava brethren, who in the *Mahābhārata* is said to have learnt the equestrian art from Droṇa. He claims to have specialized in the science and management of horses, in riding them, and in curing their ailments (*Virāṭa-parvan,* 12).

He is said to have written another work on general therapeutics, *Vaidyaka-sarvasva* (according to *Brahma-vaivarta-purāṇa*, Brahma-khaṇḍa, ch, 16), which is no longer extant. [*See* AŚVA-CHIKITSĀ].

Nāvanītaka: A compilation of medical formulae (yoga) from different ancient authorities, this text was prepared during the fourth century A.D.. Included in the *Bower*

MSs., this is the most extensive book and also the most important one in the collection. It inaugurated the long line of short manuals of formulae in Indian medicine.

It consists of seven sections, the opening section dealing with the medical uses of garlic (Laśuna-kalpa) followed by general principles (Sūtra-Sthāna), terminology (paribhāshā), and ointments for the eye and face. The second section states the purpose of this compendium, and describes the formulae in general. It claims that the important formulae prepared by great sages of yore have been included here (prākpraṇītair maharshīṇām yoga-mukhyais samanvitam). All essential medicinal preparations (pills, oils, ghee, enema, collyrium, etc.) have been listed.

The third section continues the listing of formulae while the fourth and the fifth prescribe incantations (mantra) for curative ends. The sixth treats of toxicology and gives the hymn of Mahā-māyūrī, which is further dealt with in the last section.

Written in mixed Sanskrit, the formulae are versified (in āryā, trishṭubh and anushṭubh metres). It draws extensively from Charaka and Bhela: 29 formulae from the former and 15 from the latter. There are 44 other formulae extracted from different sources like Agastya, Dhanvantari and Jīvaka (two formulae from each); Nimi, Suprabha and Kaṅkāyana (one from each); Kāśyapa (numerous formulae of his are enumerated). It is indeed a unique compilation of formulae, some of which are anonymous and not found elsewhere.

The title suggests that even as the nutritive and delicious butter (navanīta) is got by churning the curds, the helpful formulae, are extracted from numerous authorities. Explicit mention has been made of many early writers, e.g., Ātreya, Hārīta, Parāśara, Bhela, Gārga, Śāmbarya, Suśruta, Vaśishṭha, Karāla and Kāpya.

The eulogy of garlic (*laśuna*), which is not found in *CS* or *SS* (although its mention is there) is in significant detail in this work. (It can be found also in *Kāśyapa-saṁhitā* and *AHr.)* The orthodox prejudice against eating garlic has been explained here as due to its foreign origin and strong odour (na bhakshyanti enam ataś cha virprāh sanrasamparka-vinihsṛtatvāt; gandhogratām apy ata eva chāsya vadanti śāstrādhigamapravīṇāh).

This is obviously a work compiled by Buddhist enthusiasts, especially of the Mahāyāna persuasion. We find in the last two sections, incantations and hymns concerning the folk goddess incorporated into the Mahāyāna pantheon. Mahā-māyūrī. incantation has been described by the familiar tāntrik expression: 'The princess among vidyās (Ānanada-mahā-māyūrī vidyārājāya ...), uttered by the Buddha (... tathāgatabhāshitayā), for the protection (rakshā) of the patient.'

The compilation suggests the period when medicine and magic were together pressed for the patient's relief, but magic not obliterating the value of medicine: the two were independent but complementary spheres. [*See* BOWER MSs].

Nighaṇṭu: An indispensable equipment for the practising physician is an intimate acquaintance with the *Nighaṇṭu.* It is said that "the physician without *Nighaṇṭu* would come to ridicule, even as a scholar without grammar and an archer without practice."

Nighaṇṭu is vocabulary, glossary; "a collection of names" (nāma-saṁgraha), according to Hemachandra. Its original significance was a list of Vedic words (Aupamanyava and Yāska). The first *Nighaṇṭu*, on which Yāska prepared his *Nirukta*, (around 800 B.C.) comprised five sections (kāṇḍas) the first three of which dealt with synonyms, homonyms and names of deities (Naighaṇṭuka-kāṇḍa). Topics dealt with here included human anatomy and medical flora (about a hundred). Among the glossators of this Vedic *Nighaṇṭu* were SKANDA-SVĀMIN (A.D. 1060) and DEVARĀJA-YAJVA (12th century, *Nighaṇṭu nirvachana*).

The tradition of preparing glossaries was continued by Vyāḍi, Kātya, Utpala and Dhanvantari. The glossary prepared by the last alone has survived, although in a later recension known as *Dhanvantari-nighaṇṭu* (or *Dravyāvali*). It was the first medical glossary. It listed more than 370 medical flora (dravyas) and gave along with their names and synonyms brief descriptions of their pharmacological characteristics. It provided the model as well as the inspiration for later glossaries.

Amara-kośa (Nāma-liṅgānuśāsana), the celebrated lexicon prepared by AMARA-SIṀHA (5th century), in three sections (kāṇḍas), was a major achievement. The fields covered by this encyclopaedic dictionary included human anatomy, medicinal drugs and plants. But the treatment was confined to the giving of synonyms.

Medical glossaries gave not only synonyms but meanings (dravyābhidhāna) as well as pharmacological properties (dravya-guṇābhidhāna) of drugs such as chemical characteristics (guṇa), abiding taste (rasa-pradhānam āhāra-dravyam); and drug component (virya), digestive transformation of the rasa (vipāka), and the toxic effects (dosha). They also provide technical details like the terminology (paribhāshā), weight, measure and dosage (māna) of drugs, and preparations (kalpa, yoga).

The names of drugs are variously derived from convention, (rūdhi), nature (svabhāva), local usage (deśokti), external appearance (lāñchhana), resemblance (upmāna), effect (vīrya) or a deliberate naming by some one (itarāhvaya) (Rāja-nighaṇṭu). Some drugs are used as articles of food, when the main characteristic is nourishing taste (rasa-pradhānam āhāra-dravyam); and some are employed as medicines, when the systemic effect is the predominant characteristic (vīrya-pradhanam aushadha-dravyam). Others are used for their poisonous properties (visha-guṇa). Drugs are generally classified according to their food-value, curative value, nourishment value, and poisonous properties.

The essential aspects of a medical glossary would thus be pharmacological (dravya-guṇa), pathological (dosha-vaishamya) and therapeutic (chikitsā-tattva). A *nighaṇṭu* is therefore generally known as *Dravya-guṇa-saṁgraha.*

There appear to have been *nighaṇṭus* right from the days of Charaka and Suśruta; there are references to the works of Kāśyapa, Bhoja (*Abhidhāna-mañjarī*) and others in this direction, but none of them is available.

The earliest medical glossary that is extant, barring *Dhanvantari-Nighaṇṭu,* is Mādhava-kara's *Paryāya-ratna-māla* (about A.D 700), which is mainly a synonymous glossary of botanical terms useful to physicians in general. *Paryāya-muktāvalī* by HARISHEṆA is another early glossary. It is in 23 sections (vargas) dealing not only with the vegetable kingdom but with metals, minerals, precious stones and cooked food. *Sābda-chandrikā* by CHAKRAPĀṆI-DATTA (about A.D. 1060) is another medicinal glossary in nine sections dealing with herbs, minerals, alcoholic drinks, and preparations of medicines. SUREŚVARA's *Śabda-pradīpa* (about A.D. 1075) is likewise a glossary of botanical terms, the names of plants being arranged according to the divisions of vowels and consonants. The author was the court physician to a king of the Pāla dynasty, BHĪMA-PĀLA.

HEMACHANDRA (1088-1172) is the renowned author of *Abhidhāna-chintāmaṇi*, which included matter of botanical and medical interest (*Nighaṇṭu-śesha*).

Among the popular glossaries relied upon by physicians are *Soḍhala-nighaṇṭu* (12th century) following Dhanvantari, *Madana-pāla-Nighaṇṭu* (or *Madana-vinoda)* by Madana-pāla (1374), which is the most voluminous vocabulary (2,250 verses in 14 sections), *Dravya-guṇa-Śata-Ślokī,* (also called *Pathyāpathya-nighaṇṭu)* of Trimalla-bhaṭṭa (between 1383 and 1499), consisting of a hundred verses in 14 sections. *Rāja-Nighaṇṭu* (or *Abhidhāna-chūḍāmaṇi)* of Narahari (about 1400), *Śivakośa* (1677) by Śiva-datta, *Pathyāpathyavibodhaka* by Kaiya-deva (1710), *Rājavallabha-dravya-guṇa* by Rājavallabha and Nārāyaṇa-dāsa (1760), and *Paryāya-muktāvalī* by Harichandra Sena.

Celebrated manuals like *Ashṭāṅga-hṛdaya* and *Bhāva-prakāsha* were equipped with their own glossaries (*Ashṭaṅga-nighaṇṭu, Vāgbhaṭa-kośa, Bhāva-guṇa-ratna-mālā* etc.)

There are references to glossaries which are no longer available: Vopadeva's *Hṛdaya-dīpikā,* Chandra-ṇandana's *Dravya-guṇa-nighaṇṭu,* Aśoka-malla's *Nighaṇṭu-sāra* and *Abhidhāna-kośas* of Indu and Vāchaspati.

Among the recent works of this nature, the most important are *Nighaṇṭu- ratnākara, Bṛhan-Nighaṇṭu-Ratnākara, Vaidyaka-śabda-sindhu, Sālagrāma-Nighaṇṭu, Paryāyārṇava* and *Ayurveda-mahodadhi.*

There is a tendency, noticeable in more recent *nighaṇṭus,* to incorporate modern botanical knowledge (e.g., in Raghunāth Indra's *Nighaṇṭu-saṁgraha* and Virājacharaṇa Gupta's *Vanaushadhi-darpaṇa*).

There are regional preferences among physicians like *Dhanvantari-Nighaṇṭu* being popular in and around Banaras. *Bhāva-prakāsa-nighaṇṭu* and *Rāja-vallabha-nighaṇṭu* in Bengal, *Madana-pāla-nighaṇṭu* in the Hindi-speaking areas, and *Rāja-nighaṇṭu* in Mahārāshtra and Karṇāṭaka. This is not surprising because the more recent glossaries contain synonyms and explanations in the regional languages, e.g., *Śabda-chandrikā* (Bengāli), *Madana-pāla-nighaṇṭu* (Hindi) and *Rāja-nighaṇṭu* (Marāṭhi and Kannaḍa).

There is a tendency for the glossaries to increase in bulk over years, for new drugs and new properties of the old drugs are discovered, especially the drugs drawn from the vegetable kingdom. The *RV* itself contains a small nucleus of information about medical flora; the *Vedic Index* lists about 260 herbs. Kauṭilya's *Artha-śāstra* (chapters 32, 36, etc.) contains names of 330 medicinal plants. The number swells to 385 in *SS* (dravya-samgrahaṇīya section). *CS* lists about 500. *Dhanvantari-nighaṇṭu* has almost the same number (490). BHĀVA-MIŚRA provides a list of 530 plant-products (of which about 400 were of actual drug value). *Madana-pāla-nighaṇṭu* has 870, and *Nighaṇṭu-ratnākara* 820. The enlarged *Bṛhan-nighaṇṭu-ratnākara* lists over 1600 of them!

The herbal drugs known by name to the present-day physicians number about 2000, more than 500 of them being antihelminthic (kṛmināśaka). According to Śankar Dājī Sāstrī Pāde, 927 are the drugs of real value. Most of the physicians, however, work with not more than 600 drugs in all.

Nighaṇṭu-Ratnākara: A recent compilation of extracts from old and medieval medical classics, dealing with diagnosis, eight-fold clinical examination, treatment of diseases, metals and their purification, medical terminology, anatomy, preparation of decoctions and tinctures, dietetics, pharmacology and so on.

This was got compiled in three parts by V.V. GODBOLE in 1867 (Bombay), and also rendered into Marāṭhi.

Nighaṇṭu-Saṁgraha: A descriptive *materia medica* in Sanskrit prepared by RAGHUNĀTH-INDRA (Kato-bhaṭṭa) in A.D.

1893. No longer available, it is said to have contained details of as many as 607 drugs, most of which were of plant origin. (Noticed in P.V. Sharma DGV).

Nimi: He was an ancient ophthalmologist from Videha (included in the present-day Uttar Pradesh). Perhaps, he was a King, sometimes identified with Janaka. His was an honoured name in minor surgery (Śālākya-tantra). While no, work of his is available now, his views are extensively quoted in several standard medical texts. He is said to have identified 76 eye-diseases (*cf.* Ḍalhaṇa on *SS,* 6,1). He has a cure for cataract (timira): "One part of each of the following: white antimony (srotoñjana), cuttle-fish bone (sāmudra-phena), white pepper (śveta-maricha) and long pepper (pippalī); add to them one part of salt (lavaṇa) equal to an aksha (?). Powder them all finely, and this would be ideal for removing cataract" (given in *Bower MSs*).

Valuable details concerning eye-diseases can be gleaned from citations from Nimi preserved in *NiS* and *VyK* and reproduced in *HIM*, vol II, pp.339-350. [*See* DISEASES OF THE EYE].

Among the views ascribed to him, the concept of seven tastes (sweet, acid, saline, pungent, bitter, astringent and caustic: madhura-āmla-lavaṇa-kaṭu-tikta-kashāya-kshāra), the five-told classification of bodily air in terms of locations (eka eva vāyuh, sthāna-bhedāt pañchadhā), and the initial formation of the sense-organs as seats of the mind in the foetus (indriyāṇi buddhyadhisthānāni iti kṛtvā) are noticeable (*CS, Śā-Sth.* 6, 21).

P

Pālakāpya: He is the author of a comprehensive work on elephants, their diseases and treatments, *Gaja-vaidya* (according to Burnell) or *Hasti-āyurveda* (ed. Ānandāśrama Press, Poona). He is said to have been the son of a sage, SĀMAGĀYANA by name, and to have taught ROMAPĀDA, the king of Champā (or Anga?), all about elephants. Nothing more is known about the author or the time in which he lived. It does not, however, appear to be an ancient work.

The work is in four books (sthānas): Mahā-roga-sthāna (major diseases, classification of diseases, fever, tetanus, chlorosis, flatulence, fainting, diseases of the head and the foot, sweating, eye-diseases); Kshudra-roga-sthāna (minor diseases, vomiting, diarrhoea, swooning, wasting, fatigue, poisons, snake-bite, boils, erysipelas, fright, retention of urine, weakness, inflammation, wounds, prickly tongue, insanity, rheumatism, excitement, warts, ageing, colic pain, diseases of the ear, disturbances of digestion, skin diseases, and discharge of *mada* in rut); Śalya-sthāna (surgery, wounds, abscess, ulcer, fistula, sinus and their treatment, burns, bites of dogs, insects, spiders and snakes, pregnancy, difficult labour, tooth-extraction and surgical instruments); and Uttara-sthāna (supplement, oleogenous medicines, enemata, snuffs, derangement of rasas of the body, food, stables, unfavourable prognosis, expiatory rites and several recipes).

The book also deals with classification, anatomy and physiology, care and management, dietetics and complications.

Content-analysis has been provided in *HIM*, vol. II, pp.402-423.

Parāśara: An ancient sage to whom a medical work, *Parāśara-Saṁhitā*, is ascribed he was a contemporary of AGNIVEŚA. No longer extant, the work is cited by several later medical writers including ŚRĪKAṆṬHA-DATTA, ŚIVADĀSA-SENA and VIJAYA-RAKSHITA. Another work on the medicinal uses of butter-milk, Takra-kalpa, which is available, is also ascribed to him. The patient undergoing treatment by butter-milk is instructed in this work to refrain from sleep during day-time, sexual intercourse, exercise, untimely eating, untimely bath, and suppression of physiological urges (vēga-sandhāraṇā).

Some formulae, like *Parāśara-ghṛta* in tuberculosis and *Amṛtādamṛta-rasona-piṇḍa* in cases of fracture of bones and broken limbs, are ascribed to him.

There is a botanical treatise which also treats of the diseases of plants, *Vṛkshāyurveda,* which is ascribed to Parāśara. The MSs of this work was discovered by Jogendranāth Bhishagratna of Navadvīpa (Bengal), and published by his son N.N. Sircar in 1950. A work in six sections, it deals with seed formation (bījotpatti), different kinds of plants (like herbs, creepers, bushes and trees), and the treatment of plant diseases.

Paryāya-ratna-mālā: An interesting medical lexicon in 1754 verses, prepared by Mādhava-kara (7th century A.D.), the celebrated author of the *Nidāna* named after him. The main interest of this work consists in the synonyms of drugs. [*See* NIGHAṆṬU].

Pathyāpathya-vibodhaka: A descriptive pharmacological work prepared by KAIYADEVA as supplement to his own glossary of medical terms, *Nāma-ratnākara*. The date of this work is uncertain; but according to P.K. Gode, it must be prior to A.D. 1450.

The work in eight sections begins with medicinal substances and preparations (oshadhi-varga, Meharchand Lakshmandas, Lahore, 1928), followed by sections dealing with metals, cereals, drinks, preparations of food, and meat. The work closes with a miscellaneous section (miśraka-varga); and a section containing terms with multiple meanings (nānārtha-varga) has been added.

It is likely that BHĀVA-MIŚRA was acquainted with at least the first section of this work.

R

Rāja-Nighaṇṭu: Also called *Abhidhāna-chuḍāmanī,* it is an elaborate work designed to be a "compendium of the names and medicinal properties of substances" (dravyābhidhāna-guṇa-saṁgraha). The author NARAHARI hailed from Kaśmir, but appears to have lived in different parts of the country. He provides names of drugs in Sanskrit, Prākṛt and Apabhraṁśa and regional synonyms in Marāṭhī, Kannaḍa and Telugu. For description of drugs he has seven considerations: usage, effect, regional names, form, similarity, potency and place of origin. The work, as admitted by the author, follows closely the views of *Dhanvantari-nighaṇṭu (dhanvantari-matānusārakam).*

The work is in 23 sections dealing with different kinds of soil (four-fold according to caste-names, brāhmaṇa, etc, and five-fold according to the predominant *mahābhūta*), drugs, trees, fruits, metals, drinks, milk, meat, human beings, animals diseases and so on. The work was probably the first to accord the place of primal importance to pharmacology (dravya-guna). Later, pharmacology, diagnostics (nidāna), therapeutics (kāya-chikitsā), major surgery (śalya), minor surgery (śālākya), psychotherapy (bhūta-vidya), paediatrics (kaumāra-bhṛtya) and toxicology (agada-tantra) were regarded as the eight-limbs of Āyurveda.

The date of the work is hard to ascertain; but 17th century has been suggested as the probable date. The work has been printed, and is popular among physicians (Ānandāśrama, Poona 1925; and Calcutta, 1933).

Rājavallabha-Nighaṇṭu: A medical lexicon dealing with drugs and their properties relevant to the daily conduct, grouped into six sections: concerning early morning (prābhātika), late morning (paurvāhnika), noon-time (mādhyāhnika), after-noon (aparāhṇika), evening (niśābhava), and medicinal (aushadhīya) (Venkateshvara Press, Bombay, 1895).

Nothing is known about the author of this work, RĀJA-VALLABHA-VAIDYA. His date too is uncertain. But the present text has been redacted by NĀRĀYAṆA-DĀSA, whose date is given as around A.D. 1760.

Rasa-Vaiśeshika-Sūtra: A work on the basic ideas of Indian pharmacology ascribed to Nāgārjuna. It is assumed that this was the Nāgārjuna who redacted *SS*. Whatever the truth of this assumption, it is a fact that Suśruta's position agrees on essential points with the position of this work. This work has been cited frequently in Chandraṭa's *Chikitsā-kalikā*. There is a commentary on this work by Narasiṁha (Trivandrum, 1928.)

Rasāyana: The technique by which the rasa is obtained. Rasa is the essential ingredient of health and life, basic to the other constituents like blood, bone and marrow, and the source of happiness as well as the ultimate goal of life [*See* RASA]. The technique that arrests aging, wards off death, eliminates illnesses, and strengthens the sense-activities is 'Rasāyana'.

The expression is found in the early medical texts like the *CS*, *KS*, *SS*. Originally the technique consisted only of herbal formulae: "Yaj jarā-vyādhi-śamanam *aushadham* tad rasāyanam". (*Dhan. Ni.* also, *CS*, 6,1,8): but later (but not until about 1380) metals and mercurial preparations for internal and external use were prescribed.

The preparations are tonics and elixirs, especially useful in restoring the lost youth, in improving memory, sharpening intelligence, intensifying the bodily glow, strengthening the organs and securing longevity. In this sense, Rasāyana-tantra, has been included in the eight-fold (ashṭāṅga) Āyurveda. [*See* EIGHT-FOLD ĀYURVEDA]

The condition of old age is described as the diminution in the quality as well as quantity of basic fluids and tissues; and Rasāyana seeks to correct this deficiency. and restore health and vigour. Causes of old age, according to Charaka, are improper and untimely food, sleep during the day, excessive alcohol drinking, immoderate sex activity, unsuitable and abnormal exercises, and emotions like anger, fear, sorrow and greed; aging is also caused by serious disorders of body metabolism (e.g. loosening of joints of muscles, slackening of flesh, accumulation of fat, impurity of blood, decrease in bone-marrow, insufficient formation of semen, and reduction of vitality or ojas).

Several arishṭas, āsavas and rasāyanas are prescribed in the above conditions (Drākshārishṭa, Chyavana-prāśa, Amṛta-prāśa-rasāyana, etc.)

Among the exploits of the AŚVINS recounted in *RV* is the restoration of youth to the decrepit but lustful Chyavana (1.116.10: 1,117,13; 118,6., also cf. *CS*, 1,4,46

Chyavanah kāmī vṛddhah san vikṛtim gatah; vīta-varṇa-svaropetah kṛtas-tābhyām punar yuvā). *AV* also mentions the restoration of youth (rejuvenation) by drugs. Vājasaneyī-saṁhitā (12,81) speaks of four kinds of plants: somavatī (which prolongs life), aśva-vatī (which increases sexual vigour), ūrjjayantī (which increases bodily strength) and udojaśa (which gives lusture). They are described as āyur-vardhana, vājīkaraṇa, vṛshya and rasāyana respectively.

Two techniques of rasāyana are prescribed according to Vāgbhaṭa *(AHr, Utt.sth.)*: one by staying within a hut (kuṭīpraveśikam) for a prescribed period, and the other in open air (vātātapikam). Details of treatment including the drugs used are specified in early medical texts.

Rasa-Hṛdaya-Tantra: This is an old work cited by the author of *Sarva-darśana-saṁgraha,* and ascribed to BHIKSHU GOVINDA, son of SUMANO-VISHṆU, and patronised by the chieftain of the Kirāta country (Bhutān?).

In nineteen chapters (avabodha) the work deals exclusively with mercury, which it is claimed, "is the only substance that can render the body free from old age and death" (eko'sau rasa-rājah śarīram ajarāmaram kurute, 1,13). The author's aspiration is to make mankind free from poverty (nirdāridryam) and old age and death (nirjarāmaraṇam).

The author appears to be a Buddhist (cf. 19,78 Tathāgatah śreyase bhūyāt). [*See* RASA SCHOOL OF MEDICINE].

Rasa-Ratna-Samucchaya: This elaborate but anonymous work in 30 chapters deals with the Rasa school of medicine and is ascribed to VĀGBHAṬA son of SIṀHAGUPTA (sūnunā Siṁha-guptasya, 1 8), who may be different from the celebrated author of *AHr* and *AS*. The composition of this work may be placed in the 12th century.

The topics dealt with in the first ten chapters are the source, preparation, treatment and value of different kinds of mercury (rasa), cinnabar (hiṅgula), metals (gold, silver, iron, copper, zinc, tin, lead, brass), the mahā-rasas (mica or talc, turmuly, iron pyrites, fool's gold, bitumen, bismuth, calamite), the upa-rasas (sulphur, red ochre, sulphate of iron, orpiment, galena, etc.,) the sādhāraṇa-rasas (Himalayan mineral dust known as kampilla, arsenics, ammonium chloride, ambar, etc.), and precious stones.

The rest of the volume deals with diseases and treatments of diseases involving principally the rasa-drugs; fever, haemorrhagic diseases, dyspnoea, tuberculosis, vomiting, heart-diseases, piles, diarrhoea, sprue, indigestion, stranguary and other urinary disturbances, diabetes, abscess, abdominal tumour, colic pains, acidity, obesity, anaemia, skin ailments, intestinal parasites, epilepsy, insanity, ailments during pregnancy, diseases of the ear, nose, throat, fractures and cancer are extensively dealt with.

Debility, senility and loss of sexual vigour come in for elaborate consideration; treatments pertaining to rejuvenation (rasāyana) and virilification (vājīkarana) are discussed in great detail; and numerous recipes are given (chapters 26 and 27); cures for poisons of various kinds are suggested (chapter 29), and the medical value of poisons in various diseases are also indicated (29,47-159).

Of special interest are the sections dealing with the alchemical laboratory (rasa-sādhanā-rasa-śālā-rasa-maṇḍapah. 6,II-16 and rasa śālā 7,1-4), educational matters (6, 1-10), rituals connected with alchemic preparations (6, 28-42), chemical apparatus (yantra, about 40 of them, 9,3-57; crucibles of various kinds, 10, 1-31) and chemical treatments (11,1466). [*See* RASA SCHOOL OF MEDICINE]

The book is available in its entirety (Ānandāśrama Skt. Series, Pune 1890; ed. Devendranāth Sengupta, Calcutta 1915; ed, Aṁbikā-datta Śāstrī with Hindī comm. *Suratnojjvalā,* Chowkhamba Sanskrit Series, Benaras, 1939). [*See* RASA SCHOOL OF MEDICINE]

Rasārṇava: This is an anonymous work of the twelfth century, in the form of a dialogue between Pārvatī and Parameśvara. In 14 chapters (paṭalas), it deals with the chemistry and alchemy of mercurial and metallic preparations, apparatus (yantra, mūshā) and implements. [*See* THE RASA SCHOOL OF MEDICINE]

The rasa school of medicine: Two medical traditions have prevailed in the country from very early times: one is the general therapeutic complex (comprehending internal medicine and surgery), said to have been first taught by Brahmā and handed down by him through a series of teachers like Atri, Agniveśa, Charaka, Dhanvantari and Suśruta; the other is the Rasa school of medicine, first taught by Rudra and later expounded by the *Siddhas,* Chandrasena, Rāvaṇa, Māṇḍavya, Bhairava and others. Nāgārjuna's name is the only one that is included in both the lists of medical teachers. But he is more celebrated as 'Rasa-siddha'.

RUDRA, the inaugurator of the Rasa school, is celebrated as "the first of physicians" (prathamo daivyo bhishak, *YV,* 16,5) and "the best among physicians" ('bhishaktama', *RV,* 2,7,16) in the Vedic corpus (also *cf. RV,* 1,43,2 ; 1,114,1 ; 2,33,2 ; 5,42,11 ; 6,46,3 and 74,2 ; *YV,* 3,59 ; *Taittirīya-saṁhitā,* 4,5, etc). That his approach was mainly alchemic and occult becomes evident in the works ascribed to him : *Rudra-yāmala-tantra* (dealing with therapeutic uses of mercury), *Dhātu-kalpa* (medical properties of metals), *Pārada-kalpa* (preparation of mercury), *Haritāla-kalpa* (preparation of yellow orpiment) and *Abhraka-kalpa* (preparations from mica). As many as 60 mercurial preparations (rasas) are associated with his name.

The theoretical postulates of this school are close to *Śaiva-siddhānta, Raseśvara-darśana* and the *Tantras.* The legendary accounts of the life and work of 64 *siddhas* (nine among them being most famous as nava-nātha-siddhas) who lived during the early centuries of the Christian era, have contributed significantly to the celebrity of this school. Nāgārjuna is counted among these *siddhas,* and it was he who crystallized the Rasa school of thought as well as medicine.

The identity and date of this Nāgārjuna have been debated. Scholars are inclined to regard him as different from the Mādhyamaka-philospher and the redactor of *SS,* who may have lived around the beginning of the Christian era. This Nāgārjuna is specifically designated as 'Siddha-Nāgārjuna'. He is even said to have been a Jain. MERUTUṄGA refers to him as a student of the Jain master Padalipta *(Prabandha-Chintāmaṇi),* and as teacher of the king Śātavāhana of South India. al-Beruni mentions a Nāgārjuna as having lived a century prior to his visit to India (about A.D. 1000).

Whatever the position, there are books and formulae ascribed to Nāgārjuna [*See* NĀGĀRJUNA], which suggest that he was prominently involved in the popularization of the Rasa school. This school became popular in two mainstreams: one mainly alchemic (dhātu-vāda, transmutation of metals) and the other chiefly therapeutic (rasa-chikitsā, preparation of metallic and mercurial recipes for internal and external use). Nāgārjuna's name is associated with both the branches.

The traditional list of teachers of the latter branch include CHANDRASENA (sometimes regarded as the founder of the school), RĀVAṆA (king of Laṅkā), MĀṆ-

ḌAVYA, BHĀSKARA, SURASENA, KAṀBALA, VYĀḌI (the grammarian), GOVINDA, LAMPAKA and HARI. Among the authors of source-books are named RASĀṄKUŚA, BHAIRAVA, NANDI, SVACHCHHANDA-BHAIRAVA, MANTHĀNA-BHAIRAVA, KĀKA-CHAṆḌI and VĀSUDEVA *(cf. RRS)*.

Most of these are little more than names, and we do not have any books of this school that are really ancient. There is a commentary on Kaṅkāla-Rasādhyāya by Merutuñga, composed in A.D. 1386, and probably this is the oldest book on the subject that we have. *Sarva-darśana-saṁgraha* (14th century) refers to some works like *Rasārṇava* (also mentioned by *BP*), but they are not available. Among the later source-books, which represent the ascendance of the Rasa school of medicine, is *Rasa-ratna-samucchaya,* (the oldest Mss of which is dated A.D. 1699). Most of the important ideas and recipes of this school appear to have crystallized during 10th to 16th centuries.

But the foundations for the school were laid even during the Vedic times, probably earlier. The knowledge of metals was extensive and fairly accurate during the dawn of Indian civilization. The value of gold for economic, magical, and medicinal purposes was known; and the employment of metallic preparations for internal and external use was probably appreciated even then.

But classical medicine was slow to recognize the therapeutic value of metals, minerals, shells, precious stones, and chemical preparations. *CS* makes only casual references to metallic preparations involving mercury (*CS. Chi. Sth.*, 7,71). The references in *SS* are comparatively more direct (*CS, Chi, Sth.*, 25, 39). Mercurial compounds and galena or sulphide of lead (añjanā) are mentioned there, but only for external application.

It was not until the days of *BP* (about A.D. 1363) that we find the traditional physicians taking interest in mercury as a therapeutic aid. The author of *BP* was acquainted with chemical techniques (like purification of metals and calcination) and refers to several works such as *Rasārṇava, Rasa-chintāmaṇi* and *Rasa-sindhu.* From about the 15th century, the recipes involving metals and mercury began to be included in the general medical glossaries *(nighaṇṭu);* and this was probably due to Arab influence. The first to mention mercurial preparations as cures for fever, diarrhoea, jaundice, lung troubles and other diseases was *Rāja-nighaṇṭu* (13, 111). Mercury was especially prescribed for syphilis (phiraṅga) and skin ailments.

However, Indian medicine gradually tended to discourage the employment of the recipes of this school and confined its *materia medica* to the vegetable world. Nevertheless, the recipes of this school were theoretically hailed as superior to the other kinds, for in this case a small dose of medicine would be enough to cure both chronic and acute diseases, health is restored quickly, dietary regimen is unnecessary, clinical examination of the doshas and the dhātus becomes irrelevant, and consideration of seasons and places is likewise unnecessary *(Rasendra-sāra-saṁgraha).* Of the three types of treatment divine (daiva), human (mānusha) and demonic (āsura), the Rasa-medicines were included in the first group, while herbal medicine was classed under the second, and surgical operations under the third group.

Rasa, a general name for mercury, has also other meanings in the medical context: fluid, sap, flavour, taste, constituent element in the body, poison, potion, a mineral or metallic salt. In a sense, all these meanings are comprehended in the classical use of this expression. Mercury is called *rasa,* because it can liquefy all other metals (rasanāt sarva-dhātūnām), it can enhance the potency of any metal, and it can banish all ailments, prevent old age and prolong life (jarā-rug-mṛtyu-nāśāya-rasyate).

Regarded as the seed of Śiva (Hara-bîja), it occurs in five kinds: common mercury (rasa), flawless but red in colour; treated mercury (rasendra, rasa-rāja, mahā-rasa), which is brown in colour and most often used as therapeutically efficient, flawless, coarse to touch, and clear to look at; dirt-laden mercury (sūta), yellow in colour and needing the 18 chemical treatments before it can be used in medicine; extremely fluid mercury (pārada, quick-silver), white in colour and needing the treatments before it can be combined with other drugs; and mixed mercury (miśraka) with variegated colours like the peacock's tail.

Impure mercury, when used internally, can be dangerous and even fatal. The chemical treatments employed to purify mercury and render it therapeutically efficient are 18 in number (svedana, mardana, mūrchhana, uttāpana, pātana, bodhana, niyamana, dîpana, anuvāsanā, gaganādi-grāsa, garbha-druti, bāhya-druti, jāraṇa, rañjana, sāraṇa, kramaṇa, vedha and bhakshaṇa), and involve a variety of apparatus (yantras, like dolā-yantra, ūrdhvapātana-yantra, vālukāyantra, bhūdhara-yantra and svedana-yantra).

Mercury is regarded as composed of all the five elements, for it is heavy (with atomic weight of 200 and relative density being 13059, symbolising pṛthivī), fluid in normal temperature (āp), shining like molten gold (tejas), quick-moving (vāyu), and becomes invisible when heated (ākāśa). It has all the six tastes, and can set right the disorders of the three doshas, and is described as conductor of all (yoga-vāhî). Treatment of mercury is directed towards purification as well as making it therapeutically effective. According to texts, when mercury 'swoons' (mūrchchhita. viz., loses its fluidity) it can counteract all disease-conditions; when it is 'bound' (baddha, viz., assumes a gem-like shape), it produces miraculous powers; and when it is 'killed' (mṛta, viz. calcinated) it can prolong life indefinitely. Mercury in its normal condition is regarded as Brahmā; when it is bound it is likened to Vishṇu; and when it is 'killed' it is Śiva.

Usually four mercurial preparations are employed in medicine; black sulphide of mercury (kṛshṇa-bhasma or rasa-parpaṭī), the white perchloride of mercury (rasa-karpūra), the red mercurous chloride or calomel (rasa-sindhūra), and the yellow-preparation (pîta-bhasma). The most frequently employed is the red preparation.

The well-known rasa-medicines are Agni-kumāra (with mercury, sulphur, borax, opium, reduced iron and mica along with some herbs), Amṛta-kalpa (includes mercury, sulphur, borax, and Aconitum ferox), Ānanda-bhairava (includes purified cinnabar, borax and Aconitum ferox), Chaṇḍeśvara (contains mercury, sulphur, Aconitum ferox, white arsenic and reduced copper), Chandrodaya-makaradhvaja (contains red sulphide of mercury and reduced gold), Jaya-maṅgalā (contains mercury, purified sulphur, fried borax, reduced copper, tin, iron pyrites, silver and iron, and prepared gold), and Vasanta-kusumākara (contains gold, silver, tin, lead, iron, mica, coral and pearl all reduced).

This school makes extensive use of inorganic *materia medica*. Besides mercury, several metallic ores (upa-rasas), metals (dhātu), mineral salts (lavaṇa), and precious stones are used. Among metallic ores sulphur (gandhaka), mica (abhraka), iron-pyrites (svarṇa-makshika and tāra-makshika), orpiment (haritāla), realgar (manah-śilā), cinnabar (hiṅgula), bitumen with iron content (śilājit) and borax (ṭaṅkaṇa) are frequently used. The metals used include iron (lauha), gold (suvarṇa), silver (tāra), copper (tāmra), sulphate of copper (tuttha), tin (vaṅga), zinc (yaśada), lead (sîsaka), and sulphide of lead (or galena, añjanā). Alkaline ashes (kshāra), limes (śaṅkha-bhasma), arsenics (śaṅkha-visha) and red ochre (rakta-pāshāṇa, gairika) are also widely employed.

The rasa-medicines take several forms like oxides (bhasma), rasāyana, and pills (mātrā); rust or dross of iron (maṇḍūra) is commonly used as tonic. Most of the medicines are used for purposes of rejuvenation, restoration and virilification.

There are several manuals which deal with this system of medicine, many of which, however, are unpublished. Besides well-known works like *Rasendra-maṅgala* (Nāgārjuna), *Rasa-ratnākara* (Nityanātha), *Rasa-ratna-samuchchaya* (Vāgbhaṭa), and *Rasendra-sāra-saṁgraha,* there are *Rasādhyāya* (Kaṅkālaya), *Rasāyana-prakaraṇa* (Merutuṅga, 1387), *Rasa-chintāmaṇi* (Ananta-deva), *Rasa-kaumudī* (Mādhava), *Rasālaṅkāra* (Rāmeśvara), *Rasāmṛta* (Vaidyendra), *Rasa-ratna-pradīpa* (Rāma-rāja), *Rasa-rāja-Śiromaṇi* (Paraśu-rāma), *Rasa-raja-lakshmī* (Rāmeśwara), *Rasāvatāra* (Maṇikya-chandra), and other works on specific matters like *Abhraka-kalpa, Haritāla-kalpa* and *Loha-paddhati.*

Rasa-prakāśa-sudhākara: This is a comprehensive work on metals and mercury, written by YAŚODHARA from Junāgaḍh (about A.D. 1300). Opium and ambar (agnijāra) have been mentioned. Essentially a work on rasa-chemistry, but includes alchemic details also. [*See* ALCHEMY]

Rasa-ratnākara: This is a voluminous work, ascribed to NITYA-NĀTHA-SIDDHA, in five books (khaṇḍas), dealing with metallic preparations, especially mercury, for medicinal purposes.

The author claims to have consulted numerous works on the subject *(rasa-śāstra)* including the *saṁhitās, āgamas and tantras* and to have rejected everything from them excepting the really essential (tat sarvam parityajya sārabhūtam samuddṛtam). He further claims that whatever is to be found in other works can be found here, while what is to be found here cannot be found elsewhere (yad anyatra tad atrāsti, yad atrāsti na tat kvachit). The work is indeed a comprehensive one, and has been regarded as a source-book in the field.

Of the five books, the first three deal directly and extensively with medicine *(Rasa-khaṇḍa, Rasendra, vādi);* diseases and the metallic preparations indicated in them, also details like purification of metals, calcification and so on. The last two (*Rasāyana* and *Mantra*) are more concerned with alchemic, occult and spiritual matters.

The date of the work cannot be readily ascertained; however, it is later than *Rasārṇava* (13th century), which it cites [*See* RASA SCHOOL OF MEDICINE].

Rasendra-chūḍāmaṇi: A work ascribed to SOMADEVA (12-13th century), it is a comprehensive work dealing with mercury, metals and precious stones, their purification, preparation of medicinal drugs from them, laboratory techniques and implements, terminology, and the 18 classical treatments (saṁskāras) of mercury. [*See* RASA SCHOOL OF MEDICINE]

Rasendra-maṅgala: Reputed to be a work of NĀGĀRJUNA, and to be the first work in the Rasa school of Medicine, it is also called *Rasa-ratnākara.* A later work of the same name (by SIDDHA-NITYANĀTHA) recognizes this work as Nāgārjuna's (proktam Nāgārjunena yat). The work is in the nature of a conference between the King Śālivāhana, the sage Nāgārjuna and the sprite Vaṭa-yakshiṇī, and two disciples Ratna-ghosha and Māṇḍavya.

It is obviously a work of Buddhist Tantra persuasion, and contains numerous Mahāyāna ideas, especially magical conceptions.

Although the book is claimed to be

medical in intent ("vyādhitānām hitārthāya," NITYANĀṬHA), it is alchemic in content, and deals with the 18 treatments (saṁskāra), mercurial and metallic preparations, and chemical processes (ed, Jīvarām Kālidās, Goṇḍāl, 1924) [*See* NĀGĀRJUNA, ALCHEMY].

Rāvaṇa: He is the author of *Arka-prakāśa,* a work on tinctures and extracts. 'Arka' is the Sanskritized form of the Persian 'Arruck' meaning "essence." It is one of the five medicinal preparations (*dravyakalpa*), the other four being *kalka* (paste), *chūrṇa* (powder), *rasa* (expressed juice) and *taila* (oil).

The work, although ascribed to the legendary demon-king of Laṅkā, whom Rāma killed, and although written in the form of a dialogue between the demon-king and his wife Maṇḍodarī, it is clearly a work of the 16th century. It deals with opium and prescribes a preparation of mercury with śaṅkha-drāvaka for curing syphillis (phiraṅga roga), brought to India by the Portuguese. The work mentions zinc (yaśada).

There are other works ascribed to Rāvaṇa like *Kumāra-tantra* (incomplete poetical work in 201 verses, dealing with metals and their calcination), and *Nāḍī-parīkshā* (a short work in 96 verses giving the details of pulse-examination). These works also are of late origin, probably 16th century.

Ṛgveda Medicine: One of the classical Vedic triad (trayī, comprising *Ṛgveda, Yajurveda* and *Sāmaveda), Ṛgveda-Samhitā* is the only primary collection, the other two being mainly derived from it. Extant in the Śākala-recension, it is a huge mass of 1,028 hymns (sūktas) arranged in ten books (maṇḍalas) according to subjectmatter and the poet-composers. The general tenor of the Ṛgvedic collection is descriptive and laudatory, but there are interesting philosophical speculations and charming literary flourishes.

Ṛgveda is the earliest literary record of Indian culture, and it provides the common background for art, science, literature, philosophy and craft that developed in the country during the subsequent centuries. It contains a fairly elaborate account of the condition of medicine that prevailed in those days (about 7000 B.C.). It would appear that the theoretical foundations (the notions of dhātu, dosha, pañcha-bhūta, herbal medicine, nature cure, etc.), were laid even then; the essential medical practice (administration of herbal drugs, surgical operations, cure of skin ailments by sunshine, hydrotherapy, etc.) was also current.

Physicians (bhishak) belonged to a professional class. A hymn speaks of a hundred physicians and a thousand medicaments (1,24,9). The pharmacopoeia consisted mainly of herbs (oshadhī). The importance of medicinal plants (10,97,6), classification of such plants according to their therapeutic properties (10,97,110), and the collection of herbs (10,145,1) are mentioned (*cf.* also 10,19,22; 10,90,4; 10,97,4).

The Aśvins, the reputed physicians of gods, are described as custodians of herbs (10,97,110); and their skill is extensively praised (1,116,10; 1,117,13; 1,117,17; 1,112,14, etc) [*See* AŚVINS]. Among their achievements were the fitting of iron thighs (āyasīm jaṅghāṁ) to Viśpalā (wife of Khela, or a mare?) who had lost her legs in a battle (or in a race?) [1,116,15], rejuvenating the sage Chyavana who was abandoned by his people because he had grown old and infirm [1,117,13 and 5,74,5]. *Śatapatha-brāhmaṇa* 4,1,5 gives the story (*ākhyāna*)about restoration of vision to Ṛjrāśva who had become blind (1,116)

They also assisted the Vedic hero Divodāsa in his encounter with the tribal chieftain Śaṁbara (1,112,14). This Divodāsa was a physician, along with Bhāradvāja, in the *RV*. Indra's skill as a healer is also referred to (2,23,7; 2,15,7:, 8,91,7,etc.) [*See* INDRA].

Some of the gods are also healers. Sūrya, the solar divinity and the father of the Aśvins, dispels diseases (1,35,9 and 1,50,11), kills the bodily parasites (1,191,8) and eliminates the effect of poison (1,191,9, *cf.* the solar disc of Indra destroying parasites, *AV,* 2,31,1). He aids bodily secretions which contribute to activity, cheer and strength (2,38,2). Agni, the god of Fire, confers on humans long life and strength (1,12,7; 1,94,16 and 4,12,6) and prepares medicaments (6,106,3). His role as a physician is referred to in *AV* also (1,28,1). Varuṇa, the water divinity, is the lord of a thousand drugs (1,24,9). Soma, the herb, is hailed for its numerous benefits like protecting the body, removing the ailments, lifting depression, stirring good thoughts and conferring strength and cheer (6,69,7; 9,2,10; 8,48); the entire ninth book is devoted to Soma. Soma is regarded as the typical medicinal plant also in *Aitareya-brāhmaṇa* (3,40 Oshadho vai Somo). Vāstoshpati also delivers the humans from diseases.

Rudra is likewise the 'best physician'; he causes illness and cures them. But his celebrity is more apparent in *AV*. Fever (takman) and cough (*kāsikā)* are in fact his weapons (*Kau.su.,* 11,2,22 and 26); sharp pains are due to him (ibid, 31,2). Likewise, fever, (takman) is in *RV* regarded as the 'son of Varuṇa' (1,25,3; 6,96,2); dropsy (jalodara) is a disease inflicted by Varuṇa (1,25,3; 1,10,1-4).

The value of water for preserving health and removing diseases was recognised (1,23,20; 10,137,6; 6,24,2 etc.). Water contains medicine; it cures (3,12,9; 1,5,4; 3,7,5; 1,4,4): water confers deathlessness (1,25,16-24; 6,50,7; 10,9,5-7). *AV* also called it the sap of life (rasa, 3,13,5); and so does *Śatapatha-brāhmana* (3,3,3,18 raso vā āpah). Air (vāta) is also curative (1,27,3); it throws out the 'sins' from the body (10,137,2 cf. also *Taittirīya-brāhmaṇa* 2,4,1,7). Along with water and air, sunshine is recommended for health (2,33,1; 1,161,14, where 'agni' represents the Sun).

The theory of five elements being the basic constituents of the physical body is suggested (10,16,3-6). An elementary anatomy is also found (10,163; 3,36,8; 8,1,23; 6,53,8): organs like the lungs, heart, stomach, intestines, kidneys, alimentary canals are referred to. Several diseases like consumption, jaundice, heart-troubles and fevers are mentioned (10,97,105; 137,161,167, etc). Parasites (kṛmī) are recognized (1,191,1,16; 10,97,6). Difficult labour is also considered (10,172).

It is small wonder that there was a view that Āyurveda was affiliated to *RV* (Charana-vyūha, Ṛgvedasya upaveda Āyurvedah, also Nīlakaṇṭha on *Mahābhārata* 2,11,44; and *Śukranītisāra* 4,77 yasmin Ṛgvedopavedah sa chāyurveda-saṁjñakah).

Rgyud-Bzi: The most popular medical manual in Tibet and Mongolia, Rgyud-Bzi is meant to be the Tibetan rendering of a Sanskrit work of Indian origin, *Amṛta-ashṭāṅga-guhyopadeśa* (lit. Secret Teachings Concerning the Eight-fold Ambrosiac Healing). But the original has not survived; nor is there any reference to this work in subsequent medical writings. Vairochana (c. A.D. 780), the Tibetan disciple of PADMASAMBHAVA, is said to have come to India to study this text with CHANDRANANDANA (in Tibetan, Zla-ba-la dga-ba), to whom is ascribed a commentarial work *Vaidya-ashṭāṅga-vṛtti,* on Vāgbhaṭa, (cf Venkateshvara Press, Bombay, 1928, Attr with three comm.)

The work is in four parts, each called a 'treatise' (tantra): foundational (mūla), expository (ākhyāta), practical instructions (upadeśa), and supplementary (uttara). It is in the nature of a dialogue between Rig-pa'i Ye-Śes (the nirmāṇa-kāya of the Buddha as Sovereign Healer or bhaishajya-guru) and the sage Yid-las-skyes. The work has 156 chapters, and contains altogether 5900 verses.

There are several commentaries, the most important among them being *Legs-bsad-nor-bu* (in Skt. *Subhāshita-ratna*) by BYANGSPA (14th cent.) and *Vaidūrya-Sñon-po* by SDE-SANGS-RGYAS RGYA-MTSO (1635-1705). [*See* TIBETAN MEDICINE)

S

Śabda-chandriká. A medical glossary of vegetable and mineral substances, by CHAKRAPĀṆI-DATTA (*c.* A.D.1060).The work is in nine sections (vargas), dealing with trees, plants; metals like gold; and clarified butter; land, etc., human beings, animals; wines and liquors; five astringent juices (kashāya); and triphala, etc. [*See* CHAKRAPĀṆI-DATTA].

Sahadeva: He is one of the Pāṇḍava brethren, and renowned as a veterinary surgeon. A work of his, *Vyādhi-sindhu-vimardana* has been mentioned *(Brahma-vaivarta-purāṇa*, Brahma-khaṇḍa, ch.16), but is now lost.

He is celebrated as an expert in curing the diseases of cattle.

Śālagrāma-Nighaṇṭu: A modern and useful *materia medica* compiled by LĀLĀ ŚĀLA-GRĀM in 1896, to constitute the 7th and 8th chapters of *Bṛhan-nighaṇṭu-ratnākara* (*See* BṚHAN-NIGHAṆṬU-RATNĀKARA].

Śālagrāma-Nighaṇṭu-Bhūshaṇa: A pharmacological compendium prepared by Lālā Śālagrāma-Vaiśya of Moradabad in A.D. 1896 (vol. 7 and 8 of *Bṛhan-nighaṇṭu-ratnākara*, Khemraj Srikrishnadas, Bombay 1953).

The work is in two parts, the first containing 23 sections (arranged in terms of drugs, fruits, flowers, trees, metals, poisons, vegetables, drinks, milk and its products, oils, liquor, etc), and the second only two sections (kinds of soil and miscellaneous).

Although planned in the conventional style, the work includes many details of drugs of comparatively recent origin. For instance, reference to *Papaya* (Carca papaya), which is a native of Mexico and West Indies islands and came to India only with the Europeans, is to be found only here; it is called 'eraṇḍa-chirbhaṭa' in this work.

Śālihotra: A general name (Śālihotram, Śālihotrīyam) for the veterinary science concerning horses. The need to understand the nature and pedigree of horses, to manage them, care for them, and to cure their diseases was felt even during the Vedic times. We have references to animal anatomy and ailments in the Vedic texts.

But a full-fledged discipline seems to have emerged in later times, a few centuries prior to the Christian era. However, the extant works on this subject are of still later origin, several centuries after the Christian era. *Nītisāra* of Śukra is an important work, where this branch of knowledge is elaborately dealt with. The treatment of diseases of horses has been the subject-matter of several manuals, e.g., Garga's (Gaṇa's) *Aśvāyurveda* (Nepal, 765), Nakula's *Aśva-chikitsā*, Siṁha-datta's *Aśva-śāstra-samudra*, Bhoja's *Vājī-chikitsā,* Jinadatta-sūri's *Aśva-vaidyaka*, and Dīpaṁkara's *Aśva-vaidya-śāstra.*

The earliest and most comprehensive treatise on the subject was composed by ŚĀLIHOTRA of uncertain date. He is said to have been born in Śālātura in Gandhāra (the present day Kandahār), which has always been celebrated for the excellent quality of the horses bred there. His father, HAYAGHOSHA, was also an expert on horses (turaṅgama śāstra). Śālihotra is said to have learnt this art of therapeutics concerning horses from Brahmā himself, and to have written a *Saṁhitā* comprising this knowledge, at the instance of Indra (*cf.* Nakula's *Aśva-chikitsā*).

This work was composed in his own hermitage in the Champaka forest (in Magadha), on the right banks of the river Jānhavī. The work was initially known as *Turaṅga-chikitsitam* or *Hayāyurveda*, although it became famous as *Śālihotram* or *Śālihotrīya-saṁhitā*. The work mentions that Suśruta, learned in the Vedic lore, approached his father (pitaram) Śālihotra, the great sage, and requested him to give an account of the treatment of the diseases of horses (turaṅganam chikitsitam). *Agnipurāṇa* also refers to Śālihotra having taught 'hayāyurveda' to Suśruta (2, 92). This Suśruta is obviously different from the author or the first redactor of the celebrated *Suśruta-saṁhitā*.

The work is said to have consisted of 12,000 verses in eight books (sthānas). But the first book alone is available now. However, this portion contains a detailed statement of the topics dealt with in all the eight books. The chapters are entitled: Unnaya (origin, pregnancy, examination of parts, signs and characters), Uttara (diseases of horses), Śārīraka (anatomy, physiology, embryology and diseases), Chikitsitam (treatment of the colts or young ones), Uttarottara (construction of stables, rituals, pacification of evil spirits, the nīrājanā rite, worship of Revanta and Lakshmī), Siddhi (treatment of diseases), and Rahasya (duration of life, signs of death, astrological considerations, preparations and prescriptions for long life, rejuvenation, virilification, training, management, and charms).

The eight-fold character of the Indian medicine has been sought to be involved here (hayāyurveda-ashṭāṅgah). But the treatment of the subject, if we can infer from the content that is available, has not been very methodical. Diseases and treatments occur indiscriminately almost in every book.

Some specific ailments, like inability to drink fluids (sarda), prolapse of rectum (guda-bhraṁśa), facial paralysis (valardita), lameness (liṅgitāni), running from nose (siṅghāṇaka), sores within nostrils (ghṛṇī), swollen palate (avalukiravantaki), and nervous distress (vyānaka) are mentioned; probably they were described in detail.

Drugs recommended in the treatment include chebulic myrobalan (harītakī), Allium sativum (rasona), Balsamodrendron mukul (guggulu), triphala, lac (lākshā) and resin (sarjjikā). Extraction of foreign bodies, management of difficult labour, treatment of wounds and application of enemata also figure.

The supplementary section (Uttara-sthāna) is entirely magical and cultic. The next section (Siddhi-sthāna) deals with the diseases caused by the excessive use of oleogenous articles of diet, milk, wine, rice and articles like salt in food.

The available text (India Office Ms 2762) has been reproduced in *GnM, HIM,* vol.II, pp.367-372. This contains only the first book. The Mss. mentioned in *Triennial Catalogue* [Madras R. No. 2342] contains besides chapters 1 to 9 of the first book, chapters 1 to 18 of the last book. Aufrecht discovered a copy of *Śālihotra* in the East India Company library.

The work was translated into Persian during the reign of Ghiyāsuddin (Kubrat-ul-Mulk, A.D. 1381), into Tibetan (included in Tan-gyur) and into Arabic (mentioned by Haji Chalfa). The Persian translation is preserved in the Royal Library of Lucknow.

This work was abridged by King Indusena

in 1812 under the title *Sāra-saṁgraha*.

Śaraloma: He is an ancient physician quoted by Charaka as being a contemporary of Ātreya (*CS. Sū.sth.*, ch.25 Yajjah-purushīyam, 10 and 11).

In an assembly of sages in the presence of Ātreya, Vāmaka, the King of Kāśī, poses the problem of the origin of man (yajjah) and the source of disease (yajjah tasya āmayāh). On Ātreya asking the assembled sages to discuss, MAUDGALYA offered the view that soul (ātmā) being the origin of man, it was also the source of diseases (rogāś chātmajāh, kāraṇam hi sah). Diseases are occasioned by the *karma* and are meant to work it out.

Śaraloma opposes this view. Soul is the constituent of consciousness ("chetanā-dhātuh," *Chkp*) in a being, and as such it is averse to stress or misery (duhkha-dveshī). It is improbable that it would bring upon itself misery (disease) of its own accord. It is mind, being ridden by excessive activity and ignorance, although its essential nature is that of cognition and quiet (rajas tamobhyām tu manah parītam sattva-saṁjñakam), that originates the physiological constitution, and therefore it is mind that brings about ailments also (vikārāṇām cha kāraṇam).

He was the earliest thinker who suggested the psychosomatic idea of diseases.

Śārṅgadhara: He is the author of a popular medical compendium (*Saṁhitā*). He is regarded as the same as the author of the well-known literary anthology, *Śārṅgadhara-Paddhati*. The latter was the son of DĀMODARA, and grandson of RĀGHAVA-DEVA, who was minister to the Chāhuvana king Hammīra of Sākaṁbhari-deśa (Sambhal), who ruled between A.D. 1283 and 1301. The date of the anthology is given as A.D. 1363. But the medical compendium has a commentary dated *c.* A.D. 1300. It must, therefore, have been composed much earlier, and by a different author. [*See* ŚĀRṄGADHARA-SAṀHITĀ].

Śārṅgadhara-saṁhitā: This is a "short but solid text-book" (Jolly) of medical information and formulae, much relied upon by later physicians. Its composition is assigned to A.D. 1226. Little is known about the author.

The text-book is in three parts (*khaṇḍas: prathama, madhyama* and *uttara*) and 32 chapters (*adhyāya*) (7 in I, 12 in II, and 13 in III). There is a total of 2,600 verses.

Part I deals with terminology (paribhāshā), weights and measures (māna), time for taking medicine, pulse-examination (nādī-parīkshā), carminatives and stomachics, anatomy and physiology, the manner in which food is digested and assimilated in the body (āhāragati), and enumeration of well-known diseases (rogānām gaṇanā).

Part II deals with the preparation of medicines straight from plants (svarasa), decoctions (kvātha), hot infusions (phāṇṭa), cold infusions (hima), pastes (kalka), powders (chūrṇa), pills (guṭikā), lehya, electuaries, medicinal liquors (sandhāna), medicated ghees (ghṛta) and oils (taila), oxides (bhasma) of gold and other metals, purification of metals (dhātu-śuddhi) and preparation of mercurial medicines (like Vasanta-Kusumākara).

Part III details with curative procedures like oleation (snehapāna), sudation (svedana), emesis (vamana), purgation (virechana), enema therapy (basti), errhine therapy (nasya), smoking (dhūma-pāna), gargling (gaṇḍūsha), plaster (lepa), blood-letting (śoṇita-visruti), and treatment of eye-diseases.

The prescriptions are collected from numerous earlier medical works (like *CS, SS, MN, SY* and *Chakra-dattam*), but diseases are more elaborately dealt with.

The use of pulse-examination (nāḍī-parīkshā) in diagnosis appears here for the first time in medical literature. Drugs of foreign origin like opium (ahiphena) and ākārakarabha are mentioned. This is the oldest work in which calcination and similar metallurgical techniques are dealt with.

The work is frequently quoted in *BP*. There are some commentaries on it, e.g., by Vopadeva (*c.* A.D. 1300), a well-known grammarian and physician patronized by Hemādri (1260-1309) in Devagiri (modern Daulatabad, Aurangabad district, Maharashtra); by Āḍhamalla (*Dīpikā*), son of the physician Chakrapāṇi Śrīvāstavya of Mīrpur; and by Kāśīrāma (*Gūḍhārtha-dīpikā*), who was patronized by Shah Salīm, son of the Mughal monarch, Akbar.

Sarvāṅga-sundara: a commentary on *AHr* by Aruṇa-Datta (Ed. Vijaya-ratna Sen-Gupta, Calcutta, 1888, Aṇṇā Moreśhwar Kuṇṭe, Bombay 1889 along with word-index). Probably the work was written *c.* A.D. 1200. (Sarvāṅga-sundarī, according to Aufrecht's MSs and Sarvāṅga-sundara according to Hari-Śāstri Parāḍkar's MSs.)

The commentary begins with a prayer addressed to Padmanābha, and seeks to illumine the letter as well as spirit of text (*samyag-drashṭuh padārtha-bodhāya*, prefatory v.3). It is indeed an elaborate commentary, and is of immense help in understanding *AHr*. The style is lucid and engaging.

Among the medical authorities cited in this work are, besides Charaka (who is described as 'muni') and Suśruta, Agniveśa, Ātreya, Kshārapāṇi, Kāśyapa, Kharanāda, Jatūkarṇa, Bhaṭṭāra-Harichandra, Dṛḍhabala and Hārīta. The commentary refers to *AS* as 'Vṛddha-Vāgbhaṭa' (e.g., *Utt. Sth.* 36, 29 and 33) in the sense of the earlier and more elaborate work. (*See* ARUṆA-DATTA].

Śaśilekhā: This is the only commentary that is available on Vāgbhaṭa's *Ashṭāṅga-Saṁgraha* (ed. T. Rudra Paraśāva, Trichūr, Kerala, 1926). The author is INDU (or Indukara), said to be a student of Vāgbhaṭa.

Vāgbhaṭa is mentioned in this work as Bāhaṭa, a Prākrit form that became popular in the South. The commentary claims that Bāhaṭa is hard to understand, that dark is the import of his words, and that the commentary which is like the moonlight shining like a white conch (svaccha-śaṅkha-sphuta-śaśikalā), makes him lucid with words full of meaning. Hence the title "Moon's digit" (śaśi-lekhā), a reference to the author's own name Indu (meaning Moon). The commentary is quoted by Hemādri [*See* VĀGBHAṬA, ASHṬĀṄGA-SAṀGRAHA].

Śaunaka: He is an ancient sage mentioned by Charaka as having participated in the discussion on the causation of diseases (*CS, Sū. Sth.* Ch.25, Yajjah purushīyam, 26 and 27). He speaks after Kauśika who says that diseases are caused by the six constituent factors (five material elements, earth, etc., and consciousness, chetanā), even as the human constitution is.

Śaunaka argues that this would be insufficient explanation because the constituent factors by themselves do not explain the emergence of an offspring. It is heredity (parents) that is responsible for diseases, as e.g. diabetes (pitryā mehādayaś choktā rogās tāv atra kāraṇam), as also for the individual. This is the earliest reference to the diseases that are transmitted through heredity.

Śaunaka, being a family name, is borne by many ancient authors, including some medical writers. The views of the latter are quoted in manuals like *NS* and *VyKu,* but their works are no longer extant, and their identity is uncertain.

Siddha-mantra: A brief pharmacological work prepared by the physician KEŚAVA, son of MAHĀDEVA, father of the celebrated VOPADEVA (See under V), and disciple of BHĀSKARA, father of SOḌHALA, (See *S.-nighaṇṭu*). He was a resident of Vedapada on the banks of the river Varadā in the Daṇḍaka region. He was a physician to SINGHAṆA, the Yādava ruler of Devagiri (A.D. 1200-1247).

The work is so called because, as the author claims, by just repeating the recipes given here which are like well-tried *mantras*, the proper line of treatment would flash forth (sphurati bheshajam) in the mind of the physician. The work is brief in order that the physician may quickly and easily understand the principle of drugs and their qualities (sukhena drāg dravya-śakti-tattvam vidantv iti).

The work begins by propounding the fundamental principles of treatment in nine verses. The main text contains details of drugs in eight sections. The arrangement of drugs is in accordance with their effect in counteracting the doshas: vāta, pitta, kapha, vāta-pitta, kapha-vāta, kapha-pitta, dosha in general, and excess of doshas. It is interesting that the author has suggested a 'neutral' (udāsīna) group of drugs for each of the three doshas. The vāta-udāsīna drug, for instance, would neither aggravate the vāta-dosha nor counteract it. The quality, taste, potency, etc., of drug have been given in the context of the doshas.

There is a gloss on this work, entitled *Prakāśa*, by the author's son Vopadeva (See V) (*cf.* P.V. Sarma, JRIM, 1971, 6,3).

Siddha system of medicine: The use of metals, minerals and particularly mercury in medicine is an ancient practice in India. And this was a part of the Tāntric legacy inherited by Āyurveda. This legacy is conspicuous in the so-called Siddha System of medicine, which is now prevalent mostly in South India, especially in Tamil Nadu.

An old system, dating back to pre-Āyurveda period and strongly Tāntric in orientation, it got mixed up with the cult of the nine million Siddhas (nava-koṭi-siddhas). Siddhas, 'who defied death', preached a philosophy of transmuting the gross physical body composed of impure matter (aśuddhamaya) to the refined body of naturally pure matter, thereby rendering the body immutable and free from disabilities and limitations (praṇava-tanu or baindava-tanu). 'Liberated while alive' (jīvanmukta), the person who is possessed of this refined body, transacts freely with the world of impure matter as well as the world of pure matter; he is distinguished by the skills (siddhis) that facilitate these transactions.

The eighteen Siddhas (Sittars) in the Tamil tradition are as follows: Agastya (Agattiyar), Tirumūlar, Bogar, Gorakkar (Gorakshanātha), Sattai-muni, Nandīśar, Konkoṇar, Kamala-muni, Iḍaikkāḍar, Sundarāṇḍar, Roma-muni, Brahma-muni, Maccha-muni (Matsyendra?), Varāha-muni, Kūrma-muni, Punnakkisar, Kailāsa-nāthar and Kunkaṇṇar. (*cf.* A.V. Subramania Aiyar, *The Poetry and Philosophy of the Tamil Siddhas,* 1957, p. 72 fn). It is, however, doubtful if all these were historical personages.

In the classical list of Siddhas, two are of especial importance to the Tamil Siddha system. Bogar, supposed to be a pre-Christian Taoist Chinese, came to India and settled down on the Pazhani Hills in Tamilnadu. He has left not only his works on alchemy and medicine in the Tamil language but a tradition of what is known as the 'pure path' (śuddha-mārga), respected alike by the adherents of Śaivāmnāya and Śāktāmnāya.

Another Chinese who accompanied him and became an authority on medical alchemy here is known in Tamiḷ as Puḷippari. Besides these two, the name of Tirumūlar, whom tradition assigns to 3,000 B.C. (?) is associated with the founding of the Siddha school.

Agastya, an Āryan sage who came down from the Himālayan region and did his life's work in South India, is also mentioned in connection with the early development of this school. He is said to have established a centre on the Siddhakūṭa-hill in the present day Tirunelveli district in Tamiḷnāḍu. An important Tamiḷ work on which the Siddha-physicians rely is ascribed to this sage: *Agattiyar-Charakku.*

However, it is difficult to determine the origin or development of this remarkable system, especially because most of the Siddha-vaidya works in Tamiḷ have not been critically studied; very few indeed have been even published. But there is no doubt that it was once a very prevalent system. Numerous medicines, rich in mineral content, especially mercurial preparations and in extensive use today among the rural folk in the South are to be traced to this system.

The employment of mercury and arsenic as medicinal agents, extractions from minerals, preparation of essences, calcination, and the use of animal products with healing properties distinguish the Siddha practitioners. There is considerable impact of Āyurveda on the Siddha medical thought as we find it today. But this was a later development.

Of special interest in the Siddha system is the role of *muppu*, a preparation peculiar to Tamiḷ alchemy, in making mercury pills of exceedingly high potency intended to prolong life. The exact significance of the Tamiḷ expression, *muppu*, is rather obscure, but it is generally described as the Indian version of "the philosopher's stone". Its employment is twofold: transmutation of base metals to gold, and rejuvenation of the human system.

The muppu used in the Siddha system is known as the 'medicinal' one (vaidya-muppu). But another kind of muppu is employed in South Indian alchemy (vāda-muppu). Two other kinds of muppu are mentioned in Tamiḷ literature which do not appear to be substances at all; they may be mere abstractions: yoga-muppu and jñana-muppu, meant to be used exclusively by spiritual aspirants.

However, it is possible that these two kinds of muppu were psychedelic drugs, effective not only in producing visions but in stimulating the psychic centres.

There is some knowledge available about the medicinal muppu: three ingredients go into the preparation of this mixture of sodium carbonates (pūnīru), rock salt (kal-uppu), and calcium carbonate (aṇḍak-kal), which are obtained naturally. This is the substance that gives mercury its effective property; and, therefore, it is described as 'guru'.

Of the three ingredients mentioned above, important is the pūnīru (water exuded from earth). Muppu is effective in proportion to the quality of this pūnīru, which is a fluid, whitish in colour, an efflorescence from the soil. Although it is naturally got, its occurrence is restricted to certain places like Kāḷahasti, Tiruvalaṅgāḍu, Vaḍamadurai, Śivagaṅgai, Tenkāsi, Tilaivanam and Kanyākumāri.

The efflorescence, useful to a Siddha physician, is to be collected in the early hours of the morning at these places; for it is the result of the action of full moon on earth.

Tamiḷian alchemy works on the male-female (āṇ-peṇ) principle, in common with the alchemical thought in the rest of the country. The Siddha ideology looks upon the male-female symbolism in terms of bindu-nāda differentiation. Pūnīru is said to be the result of the union of male and female: full moon (male) acts on the earth (female) at some places in a peculiar way to produce this fluid. The collection is done in a ritualistic manner, and the preparation of muppu from it is even more heavily ritualistic.

There are numerous works in Tamiḷ (like

Muppuvaippu, Muppuchunnam, Pannīr-kāṇḍam, Vālaisūtram, Pacchaivettu-sūtram, Amuda-kalaijñānam) describing the several methods of muppu-preparation (bhasmam, chendūram, chunnam), but the methods are preserved as closely guarded secrets. It is necessary that the works must be carefully studied before the role of muppu in South Indian alchemy can be fully understood.

The formulary of this system includes several kinds of 'chendūram' (which, although derived from the Āyurvedic sindūram, does not always contain mercury and sulphur, nor necessarily presuppose heating to obtain sublimates), confections (lehyam, rasāyanam), pills (guḷigai, māttirai), flavoured syrups (manapāgu), different preparations of waxy consistency (mezhugu), medicated ghees, oils and butter (nei or ghṛtam, eṇṇai or tailam, veṇṇai), several kinds of calx (parapam, bhasmam), distilled essences (tīnīr) and other preparations (karpam, kalpa).

The materials used are of vegetable origin as well as metals and minerals. Drugs in powder form (chūrṇam) are mostly herbal; but the powders involving calcination (known as karuppu) contain sulphur and mercury. The coarse powders used for decoctions (Kudinīr) are again herbal, as also the linctuses (lehyam). The pills, especially the called bhairavans, may contain purified metals, minerals, and poisonous organic drugs. Sulphur; mercury; cinnabar; yellow and red orpiments; lode-stone; iron-filings; calx of mica, silver, pearls, corals, copper-pyrites; calomel; borax; aconite; opium; hemp; and biles of goat and buffalo are among the ingredients.

Nine kinds of salts (uppu), corrosive sublimates, camphor, calomel, arsenic, calx of copper-pyrites, vitriol, mercury, sulphur and cinnabar, enter into the preparation of mezhugu along with various vegetable drugs. Medicated ghees are herbal and oils are mostly herbal, although salts, calomel, borax, orpiments, musk and even mercury and sulphur are sometimes added.

The Siddha formulary is extensive; and it utilizes not only the resinous exudates, rhizomes, dried stigma (saffron), wood-barks, leaves, roots and flowers of a wide variety of plants and trees, but also animal secretions (like civet and musk), shells and bones of aquatic animals like cuttle-fish bone (samudraphena), conch-shell (śaṅkha), and oyster-shells (mauktika), horns of deer (śṛṅga), and flesh of animals.

Frequently used are, besides mercury, sulphur and cinnabar, gold, silver, zinc (jasada), lead (nāga), tin (vaṅga), mica (abhraka), red-oxide of lead (giri-sindūra), red orpiment (manahśilā), yellow orpiment (haritāla), copper-sulphate (mayūra-tutta), alum (sphaṭika), borax (ṭaṅkaṇa), calomel (rasa-karpūra, mercurous chloride), bees' wax (madhūcchishṭa) and asbestos (kalnāru). Poisons like white arsenic (śaṅkha-visha) and arsenic penta sulphide (gaurī-pāshāṇa) are also commonly included in the Siddha recipes.

This system successfully integrated the therapeutic aspects of the Rasa school with the herbal approach (kāshṭha-aushaadha) of Āyurveda. Its formulae are reputed to be remarkably effective. There is need to translate these works in Tamil concerning this system into English, so that the world may appreciate its contributions. [*See* THE RASA SCHOOL OF MEDICINE].

Siddha-yoga: A standard work on chemico-medical formulary, prepared by VṚNDA or VṚNDA-KUṆḌA (9th cent.), this is a comprehensive treatise in 82 sections (adhikāras), dealing with numerous diseases from fever to poisoning, and with elixirs and aphrodisiacs. There are accounts of the five-fold treatment procedures (bṛṁhaṇa, svedana, etc.). A section on fatal signs (arishṭa) is also included. The work recommends health-giving conduct (sad-vṛtta) and hygienic measures. The last section, miscellaneous in content, deals with the 'four-limbs' of treatment (physician, patient, medicine and nurse), weights and measures and technical terms.

The work draws heavily on *CS, SS* and *AHr.*, and appears to be modelled after *Chikitsā-kalikā*. The enumeration of diseases follows *MN*, but greater emphasis is given to curative aspects. There are many formulae included here, from his own practice and experience (siddha-yoga). Employment of metallic compounds in their medicinal preparations figures prominently. The methods for 'killing' iron, preparing sulphides of copper and mercury are given. Numerous rejuvenants and elixirs are prescribed.

Chkp has incorporated many formulae from this work in his own *Chikitsā-sāra-saṁgraha.*

It has a commentary known as *Kusumāvalī*, begun by Śrīkaṇṭha-datta (14th century) and completed by Nārāyaṇa (ed. along with *Siddhayoga*), Pune 1894 [*See* VṚNDA]

Śivadāsa-sena: He is the author of a commentary on *Chkp*, especially on *Chikitsā-saṁgraha* (Chakra-datta), entitled *Charaka-tattva-pradīpikā* and on *Dravya-guṇa-saṁgraha*. He also wrote a commentary on *AHr*, called *Tattva-bodha*.

He belonged to Bengal, and hailed from the village Malañchika (Pāvanā district, Bīrbhum). Son of Ananta-sena, a court physician of Barbak-Shāh, a chieftain of Gauḍa (1457-1474), he was patronized by this chieftain.

Śiva-kosha: Called *Nānārthaushadhi-kosha* by the author ŚIVA-DATTA-MIŚRA of the Karpūriya clan, son of Chaturbhuja-miśra, a physician, this work has become celebrated as *Śiva-kosha*, after the author. It is a pharmacological work in 540 verses, giving synonyms of drugs in alphabetical order. The work was completed in A.D. 1677 (Śaka 1599).

The author has himself written a commentary on this work, entitled *Śiva-prakāśa*, after consulting the works of Vāgbhaṭa, commentaries on them, and several pharmacological works. He has relied especially on *AHr.*

The author's son, KṚSHṆA-DATTA-MIŚRA, was also a medical writer. [*See* DRAVYA-DIPIKA].

Soḍhala-nighaṇṭu: A valuable pharmacological lexicon, prepared by SOḌHALA of Vatsa-gotra of the Rāyakavāla family, son of the physician Bhāskara who was a follower of Vāgbhaṭa, and father of the celebrated Śārṅgadeva, author of *Sangīta-ratnākara*. Besides medicine, Soḍhala was an expert in literature, grammar and astrology; he was also a poet. Another work on medicine, *Gada-nigraha*, has been ascribed to his authorship. He probably lived during the 12th century.

The work, called in the text *Nighaṇṭu-sāra-sarvasva*, follows, on the author's own admission, *Dhanvantari-nighaṇṭu* ('Dhanvantari-matoddhṛte'). The first six characteristics (lakshaṇa), and the eighth deals with various articles of food with medicinal properties: drinks, milk, butter, butter-milk, ghee, oils, sugar-cane, honey, liquors, urine, etc. The last subsection (27th) is miscellaneous (miśrakādhyāya). At the end is given details of drugs like taste, potency etc., following *AHr.*

The work refers to mercury (pārada) and the processes to make it effective. But there is no mention of zinc (yaśada) among metals, nor of opium, bhaṅg and Ākarakara.

Śrīkaṇṭha-datta: He is the author of *Madhu-Kosha* (along with VIJAYA-RAKSHITA) a commentary on *MN*, from the section on urinary disorders (prameha, 33) till the end.

It is a work of the 13th century.

Son of Nārāyaṇa, he studied medicine under Vijaya-Rakshita, and completed the commentary that his teacher had begun on *MN* and left unfinished at the end of the section on calculus (*aśmarī,* 32). He has two verses before the commentary on the section 33, wherein he tells us that his commentary was motivated by his reverence for the teacher Vijaya (Śrīkaṇṭha-datta-bhishajā guru-bhakti-leśād-ārabhyate ...).

At the close of the commentary he refers to his teacher's work, *Sūkti-muktāvalī* (which probably is another name for *Madhu-Kośa*), in which whatever was left unarticulated by his teacher (guruṇā yan na gumphitam) has been supplied by himself in the very words of his teacher (mayā samastam agranthi tad girā śuddhi-yuktayā).

He also wrote a learned commentary on *SY.* [*See* MADHU-KOŚA AND VIJAYA-RAKSHITA].

Suśruta: Author or first redactor of the well-known book on surgery, *Suśruta-Saṁhitā,* he is said to have learnt the art and science of surgery from Dhanvantari (-Divodāsa) in the Himālayan retreat, along with other sages (Aupadhenava, Vaitaraṇa, Aurabhra, Paushkalāvata, Karavīrya and Gopura-rakshita) (*SS*, 1, 1 and 5, 2). The author of *SS* refers to Śusruta in the third person, and describes him as the worthy son of Viśvāmitra (Viśvāmitra-sutah śrīmān Suśrutah) (*SS, Utt. Sth.* 66, also *Chik. Sth.*, 2).

It is difficult to identify who this Viśvāmitra was, for Viśvāmitra is a family name. The original Viśvāmitra (the gotra originator), is a ṚgVedic sage, the author of the celebrated gāyatrī hymn. He is described as the son of Kuśika (or Gādhi), the King of Kānyakubja, and as the family priest of the King Sudāsa. There is a Viśvāmitra, a descendent of his, who was a physician and whom *Nis, VyK, VyMk* and *BP* quote. Suśruta was probably the son of this Viśvāmitra.

There seems to have been a Suśruta in ancient times, probably a contemporary of Agniveśa, and long before the redaction of the present *SS*. He is referred to as Vṛddha-Suśruta, and is described as the author of a medical work (*tantra*). *NiS, VyMk, BP, Toḍarānanda* and *Tattva-chandrikā* quote from this work (*Sauśruta-tantra)*. The expression 'Sauśruta' here is explained as 'taught by Suśruta' in the *Vārttika* of Kātyāyana, 4th century B.C. Perhaps it is this ancient Suśruta, who is saluted in the beginning of *SS* along with the ancient teachers of medicine in succession (namo Brahma-Prajāpaty-śvinā-Balabhid-Dhanvantari-Suśruta-prabhṛtibhyah). It may be noticed that *Bower MSs*(*Nāvanīta-ka*) refers to Suśruta as a sage (ṛshi), while it does not mention Charaka at all.

It may be presumed that the original *Saṁhitā* according to Dhanvantari-Divodāsa's teachings was the work of this elder Suśrutā, who may have lived before or around B.C. 600 (as Hoernle supposed), or even about B.C. 1000 (as G.N. Mukhopadhyaya held). The work was probably recast at a later date, in the early century of the Christian era.

There is a Suśruta who is referred to as the court-physician of Kanishka (whose date is variously given between A.D. 78 and 144) and another in the court of Yaśovarman of Kānyakubja (A.D. 899-910). It may be the former who gave *SS* the present shape. [*See* SUŚRUTA-SAṀHITĀ].

Suśruta-Samhitā: A work comprehending the surgical tradition of Indian medicine, ascribed to the sage Suśruta, the original of which may have been composed around 600 B.C. (Hoernle) or before 1000 B.C. (G.N. Mukhopadhyaya). It was one of the four treatises regarded as the source-books for the branch of surgery and for all the later surgical works in India (śeshānām śalyatantrāṇām mūlam etāni, SS, 1, 4). The other three (Aupadhenava, Aurabhra, and Paushkalāvaṭa) being no longer extant, this one (Sauśruta) has an added importance.

It is unlikely that the present *SS* is the original one; it may have been redacted by another Suśruta in the first century A.D.. The text claims to contain the teachings of Dhanvantari in one of the eight branches of medicine, viz., surgery (śalya). The chapters begin with "As the revered Dhanvantari taught Suśruta" (yathovācha bhagavān Dhanvantarih Suśrutāya). The followers of Dhanvantari (called Dhānvantarīyas) were popular even during the days of Charaka as specialists in surgical operations (*CS, Chik.* Sth. 5, tatra Dhānvantarīyāṇām adhikārah kriyāvidhau; vaidyānām kṛta-yogānām vyadha-śodhana-ropaṇe).

Ḍalhaṇa, the celebrated commentator on *SS*, mentions that *SS* was redacted by Nāgārjuna (prati-saṁskarttā'pīha Nāgārjuna eva, *SS*, 1,1). The Nāgārjuna that is referred to here may have been the great Mahāyāna master and alchemist who lived in the first century A.D. [*See* NĀGĀRJUNA].

Thus the extant *SS* has three layers: the original treatise by the 'elder' Suśruta (*Vṛddha-Suśruta*), the later recasting by Suśruta, and the still later additions and amendments by Nāgārjuna. But it is impossible to segregate them in the present corpus of *SS*. However, the last book (*Uttara-tantra*), which is in the form of a supplementary section, is decidedly a later addition.

The extant *SS* consists of six books (sthānas) and 184 chapters (adhyāya). But it was obvious that the original *Saṁhitā* consisted only of five books and 120 chapters. The content scheme provided in *SS, Sū. Sth.* 3, gives this number (sa-viṁśam adhyāya-śatam pañchasu sthāneshu), as well as the break-down: 46 chapters in Book 1 (*Sūtra-Sthāna*), 16 in Bk II (*Nidāna-Sthāna*), 10 in Bk III (*Śārīra-Sthāna*), 40 in Bk IV (*Chikitsā-Sthāna*), and 8 in Bk V (*Kalpa-Sthāna*). Descriptive titles are also given here.

After the enumeration of the eight chapters in Book I, thus drawing the section on contents to a close (adhyāyānām śatam viṁśam evam udīritam), there is a half-verse (29) which introduces the sixth Book (uttara-tantra): "Hereafter (atah-param) the later section (tantram uttaram), by its very name as later (sva-nāmnaiva), will be described".

While the first five Books deal almost extensively with surgery (*śalya*), the last Book (supplementary) is designed to deal briefly with the other six branches of Āyurveda (śālākya-tantra, kumāra-tantra, kāya-tantra, bhūta-tantra, rasāyana and vājīkaraṇa), leaving out toxicology (agada-tantra). The expression uttara is explained as 'the best' (śreshthatvād), 'the section that deals with many matters' (bahvartha-saṁgrahāt), or the section which comes at the end, viz. after the main thing is discussed' (paśchimam) (v. 43).

Book I (*Sūtra-Sthāna*) (46 chapters) deals with preliminary matters concerning medical study. It provides the framework of surgery as the focal theme of the work. Surgical instruments are described, and instructions regarding operations are given. 'Śalya' is defined in terms of extraneous matter that is introduced into the body. Diseases are classified, and prognostic details are mentioned. The rôle of the three dhātus (vāta, pitta and kapha) is explained. Drugs are classified, and their curative merits (like emetic, purgative, alterative, etc.) specified.

Interesting aspects of this book which can be called the 'First Principles' are the introduction to medical science (especially surgery), medical education and training, the theory of therapeutic substances, and dietetics.

Book 2 deals with pathology (*Nidāna-Sthāna*) (16 chapters), causes and symptoms of various diseases (diseases of the nervous system, haemorrhoids, calculus in bladder, fistula-in-ano, diseases of the skin, urinary ailments, abdominal tumours, dropsy, internal abscess, enlargement of glands and of scrotum, venereal diseases, elephantiasis, fractures and dislocations and diseases of the mouth.

Book 3 (*Śārīra-Sthāna*) (10 chapters), is mainly devoted to anatomy and physiology. But the human constitution is also explained with reference to the 'soul' and foetal growth. Vital parts of the body (marma-sthānas), the vascular system, venesection, management of pregnancy and handling of children have been explained.

Book 4 (*Chikitsā-Sthāna*) (40 chapters) is an elaborate account of therapeutics in various diseases. Ulcers, wounds, haemorrhoids and fractures are dealt with first, and are followed by other ailments (like skin-diseases, urinary disorders, diabetes and abscesses, diseases of the mouth, and swellings). Preventive medicine is considered next, followed by prescriptions of standard formulae. Rejuvenation and virilification are also dealt with here. Medicated oils and baths, emetics, purgatives, syringes, enema, inhalations and gargles constitute the closing of the Book.

Book 5 (*Kalpa-Sthāna*) (8 chapters) deals with vegetable, mineral and animal poisons. The chapter opens with possible food poisons, and goes on to deal with snake-bites, bites of other animals like rats, dogs and jackals. Treatment and drugs are also prescribed. The chapter closes with insect-bites.

An interesting and intriguing detail to be found in this Book is the suggestion that loud sounds of the drum (dundubhi) smeared with antidotes are capable of destroying poisonous germs that float in the air (bheryah paṭahaścha digdhā nānadyamānā visham āśu hanyuh, 7, 72). Hearing these sounds, or looking at the flags and festoons smeared with the antidotes or touching them prevent the contagion of poison (śravaṇād darśanāt sparśāt vishāt saṃpratimuchyate).

The supplementary Book (uttara-tantra), which is voluminous (66 chapters) is now regarded as Book 6. In the first division (26 chapters) pertaining to minor surgery (śālākya) (19 chapters) deal with diseases of the eye and their treatment. The next two chapters are devoted to the diseases of the ears, the next three to the diseases of the nose, and the last two to diseases of the head. This is followed by the division (12 chapters) pertaining to paediatrics. Along with the diseases that affect the children (kumāra-tantra) influence of evil spirits (seizures, *graha*) is also dealt with. The third division (21 chapters), general therapeutics (*kāya-chikitsā*), deals with fever, diarrhoea, consumption, tumours, heart-diseases, anaemia, jaundice, haemorrhage, fainting, alcoholism, asthma, dysuria and strangury. The fourth division (three chapters) deals with insanity and epilepsy with reference to supernatural aetiology (thus called bhūta-vidyā-tantra) as well as with normal medical aspects. The final division of the section (four chapters) is general in nature, dealing with the six tastes (rasa), principles of hygiene, medical terminology and the abnormal operations of the doshas.

The *SS* is remarkable in many respects. As many as 76 kinds of eye-diseases are described, of which 51 are regarded as cases for ophthalmic surgery. It deals with cataract-crouching. The author was aware of the optical lense being the seat of vision. [*See* OPHTHALMOLOGY]. The work describes 101 blunt instruments and 20 sharp instruments suitable for surgery; the former group includes various pincers, forceps, hooks, tubes, etc., and the latter, many cutting devices like knives, scissors, bistouries, lancets, saws, trocars and needles. Different kinds of operations like excision, incision, scarification, puncture, probing, drainage of fluids, and suturing are described. [*See* SURGICAL INSTRUMENTS].

Operative treatment of harelip, rhinoplasty, herniotomy, laparatomy, extirpation of tumours, removal of ovaries and fistula are dealt with. Midwifery is a special area of the medical care and treatment that is elaborated here. Application of forceps and Caesarean section in cases of difficult delivery are suggested here. [*See* MIDWIFERY].

As many as 300 surgical operations (with 42 different surgical processes) are considered here. The amputation of limbs, setting of fractures, abdominal sections, treatment of splenic enlargement, removal of fistula and haemorrhoids, reduction of hernia and ruptures, and obstetric manipulation are some of the surgical problems that have been attended to. Fourteen kinds of dressings are discussed here [*See* SURGERY].

The work describes 12 kinds of leeches (six of which are poisonous) for purposes of blood-letting.

SS deals with 1,120 diseases, grouped under three heads: bodily ailments due to injury; natural infirmities due to old age (including congenital diseases); and mental disorders. It mentions over 700 plants of medicinal value, and also classifies them into 37 groups (*gaṇas*) of diseases in which they are indicated.

It may be noted that the vegetable drugs prescribed here are larger in number than what we find in *CS*; and the drugs of animal origin are less in number (177 in *CS*, 57 in *SS*), while the number of minerals and metals used as drugs remains the same in both (64).

The work was translated into Arabic even before the 8th century closed. Known as *Kitab-Shah-Shun-al-Hindi*, it was rendered from the original Sanskrit into Arabic by Ibn Abillsaibial. It was also known as *The Book of Suśruta (Kitab-i-Suśrud)*. Rhazes (b. A.D. 680) was acquainted with *SS*.

Among the early editions of *SS* Madhusūdan Datta's (Calcutta 1835), Jībānanda Vidyāsāgar's (Calcutta 1877), and Avināshchandra Kaviratna's (Calcutta 1888) are prominent. The work was translated into English in parts by U.C. Datta (1883), A. Chaṭṭopādhyāya (1891), A.F.R. Hoernle (1897) and the complete translation was done by A.M. Kuṇṭe (Bombay 1876) and Kuñja-lāl Bhishagratna (1907-11).
Hessler's Latin translation is not available now.

The text of *SS* appears to have had many readings, as can be gleaned from the commentary of Jaijjaṭa, Ḍalhaṇa and *Chkp* (*Bhānumatī*). Chandraṭa, son of Tīsaṭa, attempted to restore the original reading (Suśrute pāṭhaśuddhim Chandraṭo vyadhāt); but the work is no longer available.

There are two epitomes of *SS*, *Laghu-Suśruta* and *Suśruta-Sāra*.

The earliest commentary on *SS* was by Jaijjaṭa, whom the well-known gloss *NiS* quotes. The work has unfortunately not come down to us. There is an incomplete commentary by Gayadāsa (10th century?), known as *Nyāya-chandrikā* (or *Sauśruta-pañjikā*), also quoted in *NiS* frequently. There is another incomplete commentary (till *SS*, 1,43,5) by Chakrapāṇi-Datta, the celebrated commentator on *CS* (*c*.1060), called Bhānumatī (or *Tātparyaṭīkā*) (ed. by Gaṅgāprasād Sen, along with *NiS*, Calcutta 1888). Brahma-deva (*c*. A.D. 1080) wrote a gloss (*ṭippaṇa*) on *SS*, which also has been referred to in *NiS*. Gadādhara, father of Vaṅga-sena, is said to have compiled a metrical summary of *SS* (Suśruta-śloka-vārttika-praśna-vidhāna-ṭīkā), which has been cited in *VyMK*. There are references to two other commentaries by Bhāskara and Mādhava.

The most important commentary, however, is *Nibandha-saṁgraha* by Ḍalhaṇa (12th century) (ed. by Gaṅgāprasād Sen, in 15 parts, Calcutta 1888 onwards; Jībānanda

Vidyāsāgara, Calcutta 1891; Avināsh Chandra Kaviratna and Chandra Kumār Gupta, Calcutta 1885 onwards). It utilizes the earlier commentaries by Jaijjaṭa, Bhāskara, Mādhava, Gayadāsa and Brahma-deva. It quotes another commentary *Gūḍha-pada-bhaṅga-ṭippaṇa* of unknown authorship *[See* ḌALHAṆA].

T

Tibetan medicine: When Tibetan religion and way of life were Indianised during the seventh century, Indian medicine also made a formal entry into this Himālayan region. It is probable that the folk practices in all the Himālayan countries were common, and therefore considerable medical wisdom must have been included in the transaction between the Indian side of the Himalayas and the Tibetan.

It is, however, uncertain what the state of Tibetan medicine was like during the days when Bon religion alone prevailed. But many of the practices characteristic of this period survived in later Tibetan medicine. Important among them are protective charms (shu-deg, Yungs-kar, etc.), talismans worn about the neck or tied round the arms, precious stones and minerals, mystic pills often containing mercury (rin-chen ril-bu), and employment of shamans to drive away the demon of disease by incantations and awesome ritual. It may be noted that such practices were prevalent in India also at that time, and that they have survived to this day.

Tibetan medicine accepted the basic principles (e.g. the pāñcha-bhautika theory, the tri-dosha doctrine, the concept of preventive medicine) and practices (herbal medicine, rasāyana, diagnosis and prognosis, diet, regimen, etc.) of Āyurveda and adapted them to the geographical and cultural conditions peculiar to Tibet. Thus, there are aspects of Tibetan medicine which have grown beyond the confines of Āyurveda (like pulse-examination and urine examination), and which contain the hard core of local folk practices. Unfortunately, the world is as yet little acquainted with all the dimensions of Tibetan medicine, despite some valuable publications in English in this field (e.g., *Principles of Lamaist Pharmacognosy* by Brtan-dzan-phun-tshogs, Leh, 1970; *An illustrated Tibeto-Mongolian Materia Medica of Āyurveda* by Lokesh-Chandra, New Delhi, 1971; *Tibetan Medicine* by Rechung Rimpche, Berkeley, Univ. of California Press, 1973; *Tibetan Medicine with special reference to Yoga-Śataka*, by Bhagwan Dash, Library of Tibetan Works and Archives, Daramsala, India, 1976; *The Ambrosia Heart Tantra,* with annotations by Yeshi Doenden, Tr. by Jhampa Kelsana, Library of Tibetan Works and Archives, 1977.

These and other texts were cast from Sanskrit into Tibetan by official translators (lo-tsā-ba) during the reigns of the Tibetan Kings Khri-Srong-lde-btsan and Ral-pa-chan (between A.D. 750 and 836). Many more Indian works of medicine arrived in Tibet during the reign of Ye-Śes-'od in the 10th century. Tibetan medicine may be said to have assumed its present form (based largely on Āyurveda) during the period between the 12th and the 14th centuries. Medicine was accorded a place in the traditional five-fold 'branches of learning' (rig-gnas, skt. vidyā-sthāna), as gso-ba-rig-pa (i.e., *chikitsā-śastra*), other four being arts and crafts, *bzn-rig-pa*, grammar and prosody, *Sgra'i-rig-pa,* logic and the art of exposition and disputation, *tshad-ma-rig-pa,* and religious studies. *man-doṅ-rig-pa.*

Tibetan translations of Sanskrit texts on medicine along with their commentaries in Tibetan were included in one of the two sacred canons of Tibetan Buddhism, viz. Bstan-hgyur (the Tanjūr). There are as many as 22 medical texts of Indian origin included in this collection (to be found in volumes Se, He, E, Ko, Kho, No, Mo and Do of the Narthang edition). These works are valuable inasmuch as their original Sanskrit versions have been lost in most cases, almost irretrievably, e.g., Nāgārjuna's *Vaidyajīva-sūtra,* Chandranandana's *Aṣṭāṅga-hṛdaya-vṛtti* and *Padārtha-Chandrikā* (another commentary on Vāgbhaṭa's work), Ravigupta's *Vaidya-siddha-sāra,* Dānadāsa's *Bheshaja-saṁskāra,* Vyāḍi's *Rasāyana-Śāstroddhṛti,* and Raghunātha's (described as a Kshatriya of Mathurā in the Magadha country) *Bhishak-Raghunāthāmnāya*).

The most popular among such works, and most often relied upon by medical practitioners in Tibet, is *Rgyud-bźi,* whose title in Sanskrit is given as *Amṛta-aṣhṭāṅga-guhyopadeśa.* Legend relates that the Indian patriarch in Tibet, Padmasaṁbhava (to whom the entire Lāmāist system is due), directed his Tibetan disciple Vairochana to go to India and learn this text from the then celebrated physician in India, Chandranandana (Zla-ba-la-dga-ba in Tibetan), around A.D. 780. Ascribed to this Indian teacher of medicine is a gloss on Vāgbhaṭa known as *Vaidya-ashṭāṅga-hṛdaya-vṛtti,* (*cf. AHr* edition by Venkateśhwar Press, Bombay, 1928) the Tibetan translation of which has been preserved. In the 10th century, another Tibetan of note, Rin-Chen bzang-po, came to India and lived here for ten years studying medicine according to Vāgbhaṭa's system.

As in Āyurveda in India, in Tibetan medicine also Charaka, Suśruta and Vāgbhaṭa have provided the main framework. If the lineage of medical masters in India begins with Brahmā the creator, the Tibetan lineage begins with Buddha-Kāśyapa who taught Brahmā, who in turn taught Daksha-prajāpati.

The patron-deity of medicine as well the progenitor of the medical system in Tibet is the Buddha-Śākyamuni as 'Sovereign Healer', who in his *saṁbhoga-kāya* appears with his right hand held in a gesture of assurance (*abhaya*) and also holding a fruit of myrobalan (regarded as the most effective drug), and his left hand holding a bowl containing three kinds of 'ambrosia' or remedies, one for combating ailments and driving away death, the second for combating the ill-effects of age, and the third for invigorating the mind and facilitating meditative absorption. He is said to have delivered not only the medical teaachings but the most effective formulae for curing 404 ailments.

The subsequent succession of medical teachers is the same in both accounts: Aśvins, Indra and Atreya. In the Tibetan account Atreya's line continues through DKa-'gnis spyod, Mu-khyud-'dzin, Gshol 'gro sKyed, Me-bźin-'jug (Agniveśa), Lug-nag (*Kṛishṇa-meṣha?*) and Raya-skegs sña. Each of these wrote a treatise, and all the works were compiled and redacted by Rtsa-ra-ka (viz., Charaka). This work is known as Rtsa-ra-ka sde brgyud (in Skt. *Charaka-aṣhṭavarga*). There is an elaborate Tibetan commentary on this work by the sage Ldan-'phreng-ba, running to about 600 chapters.

Atreya is also regarded as the teacher of Thang-la-'bar (viz., Dhanvantari), from whom the surgical system evolved. It would appear that surgery was at one time practised in Tibet; but it was abandoned in due course, and does not figure in the present-day Tibetan medicine.

It is probable that alchemy was an aspect of medicine even in pre-Buddhist Tibet. But its importance grew due to the impact of

Nāgārjuna (in Tibetan, Klu-grub), the great versatile genius whose works on varied subjects number about 200 in their Tibetan translations. In Tibet, his fame rests not only as a philosopher and as a tāntrik but also as an alchemist (*rasa-siddha*) and as a medical author (*See* NĀGĀRJUNA). There are many works in Tibetan on the employment of mercury in medicine, some of which are ascribed to Nāgārjuna. The concept of ambrosia (*amṛta*), actually an alchemic preparation meant to conquer death and diseases (404 ailments), in involved in the Tibetan medical lore in a significant manner.

Although Āyurveda provided Tibetan medicine with the basic conceptual framework and the essential pharmacopoea, Tibetan genius made many innovations and discovered numerous indigenous drugs. Of great importance are the methods of examination of pulse and urine, that were remarkably efficient as diagnostic aids among the traditional medical practitioners in Tibet (known as *emchis*).

Tīsaṭa: He is the author of *Chikitsā-kalikā*, a popular medical work of 400 verses composed during the Gupta period (*c.* A.D. 500). It was intended mainly for the student of medicine.

The name suggests the author's Kāshmīri origin. One of the MSs. mentions that he was Vāgbhaṭa's son, but this appears to be a mistake.

His son, Chandraṭa, was also a medical writer. [*See* CHIKITSĀ-KALIKĀ].

Toḍarānanda: This is a comprehensive compendium of general information got prepared by Toḍara-malla (around 1589), a khatrī nobleman from Punjāb and minister of the Mughal emperor, Akbar. It includes an extensive medical work known as *Āyurveda-saukhyam* (Anūp Skt. Lib., Bikaner). Several experts from Banaras are said to have contributed to this gigantic work, dealing with 23 different aspects of traditional culture, including medicine.

Āyurveda-saukhyam is encyclopaedic in its nature, and comprises 97 chapters, dealing with the basic principles, *materia medica (nighaṇṭu)*, iatro-chemistry, pathology and examination, treatment of diseases and hygiene. The voluminous work is still unpublished in its entirety. The portions (10) dealing with drugs of vegetable, mineral and animal origin (*materia medica*) have been collected, edited and translated into English by Bhagavān Dāsh and Lalitesh Kāshyap in a volume (*Materia Medica of Ayurveda* , Concept Puhlishing Co., New Delhi, 1979). The first six chapters of the work have been planned to be brought out in another volume (*Basic Principles of Ayurveda*) by the same authors.

Verses from *BP* are found to be included in this work. There is a suggestion that Bhāva-Miśra was associated with Toḍara-malla's project.

U

Urgāditya: Author of *Kalyāṇa-kāraka* (*c.* A.D. 850), this Jaina ascetic belonged to the Deśī-gaṇa, Pustaka-gaccha of the Panaśoka (the present-day Hanasoge village in Mysore district in Karṇāṭaka) branch of the Mūla-saṁgha in the lineage of the celebrated Kundakunda.

He learnt medicine under another Jaina teacher Śrī-nandi who resided on the mount Rāma-giri in Trikaliṅga-deśa identified with the modern Rāma-tīrtha or Ramakoṇḍa in

Viśākhapaṭṭaṇam District in Āndhra Pradesh. This work was written on the same mount.

He is said to have visited the court of the Rāshṭrakūṭa monarch, Nṛpatuṅga-Amoghavarsha I (A.D. 815-877) of Mānyakheṭa to deliver a discourse on the need to reject the use of animal food in medicine (vaidya-śāstreshu māṁsanirākaraṇārtham). This discourse has been included as an addendum (pariśishṭa) to *Kalyāṇa-kāraka*, entitled *Hitāhitādhyāya* (the section on what is good and bad for health). He also argues against the use of alcoholic preparations for medicine. [*See* KALYĀṆA-KĀRAKA].

V

Vāgbhaṭa: Regarded as the author of one of the three major medical source-books (*saṁhitā*) in India, he is classed with Charaka and Suśruta, and held in great reverence all over India, especially in the South.

While Indian tradition is acquainted with but one Vāgbhaṭa, the author of two treatises *Aṣṭāṅga-saṁgraha (AS)* and *Ashtāṅga-hṛdaya-saṁhitā (AHr)* based on the former, Hoernle argued that the author of the former work was Vāgbhaṭa I (Vṛddha-Vāgbhaṭa) who lived in the 7th century (A.D. 625); and that the author of the other work was Vāgbhaṭa II, who perhaps lived a century later (*Medicine in Ancient India,* pp. 10-15). Although his evidence was slender and far-fetched his views have been widely accepted even by Indian scholars. But Gn. Sen and Hari-Śāstrī Parāḍkar have conclusively proved that the traditional view of one Vāgbhaṭa is valid. The numerous commentators on *AHr* as well as all later medical writers in India have always held this view.

Vāgbhaṭa, son of Siṁhagupta was named after his grandfather, the great physician Vāgbhaṭa (bhishagvaro Vāgbhaṭa ity abhūn me pitāmaho, nāma-dharo'smi yasya); he hailed from the Sindhū country (Sind). He studied medicine under his own father, and later under a Buddhist mendicant and physician, Avalokita by name (samādhigamya guror Avalokitāt). He himself recounts that he "churned the ocean of Indian medicine with its eight divisions and prepared *AS*", which was an immense work; and that finding it unwieldy for general practitioners and students, he abridged it in *AHr.*

The former work is not only voluminous but is in mixed prose and verse, as *CS* and *SS* are, while the latter is shorter and is versified, often with considerable poetic flourish, so that students would find it easy to memorize. The contents and literary style leave no doubt that author of the two works was the same. The former is usually referred to as Vṛddha-Vāgbhaṭa (meaning 'elaborate') and included in the 'Big Three' (*Vṛddha-trayī*) of Āyurveda; and the latter, called Laghu-Vāgbhaṭa (meaning 'concise') is included in the 'Little Three' (*Laghu-trayī*).

Gn. Sen assigns him to fifth century A.D. on the basis of the possible reference to Vāgbhaṭa by the Chinese pilgrim, I-tsing, when he said that originally medicine existed in India in eight books, and that lately they were compiled in one book by an author (*Records*, Takakusu, p.128). Hari-Śāstrī Parāḍkar, the editor of the standard text of *AHr*, holds that he belonged to the latter half of the fourth century on several considerations (Skt. Intro. p.15). Kuṇṭe would push his date back to the first or second century B.C. . Hoernle, who had two Vāgbhaṭas in his mind, placed Vāgbhaṭa I around A.D. 625(*Osteology,* Oxford, Intro. p.11) and Vāgbhaṭa II in the 8th or 9th century (Ibid., p.16).

Reference to Buddhist religion are numerous in his two books, and it is likely that he was a Buddhist. The name of his teacher (Avalokita) certainly suggests that he was a Buddhist. Devotion to divinities like Ārya-Avalokita, Parṇa-Śabarī, Aparājitā, Maha-māyūri and Ārya-Tārā (who are of folk origin but were assimilated into the Buddhist pantheon) is prescribed as a curative aid (*Chik.* 2). Some spells which are typically Buddhist (*dhārnaṇīs*) are also mentioned. His manner of dedicating the merit he acquires by writing this work to the weal and welfare of all beings is also characteristically Buddhist (kṛtvā yach chubhaṁ āptam śubham astu tato jagatah *AHr.*, 3,40,9).

However, that he was not a dogmatic Buddhist and that he was favourably inclined towards the Vedic culture also are amply evidenced in his books (*cf.* A.M. Kuṇṭe: *Intro. AHr.* 1880, pp.5-6).

Among his students Indu and Jaijjaṭa are counted. The former has prepared a commentary entitled *Śaśilekha* on *AS*, the only commentary available on it.

There are several other Vāgbhaṭas known to Indian literature, including the one who wrote *Rasa-ratna-samuchchaya*, a work of the thirteenth century prescribing mineral recipes for diseases [*See* ASHṬĀṄGA-HṚDAYA and ASHṬĀṄGA-SAṀGRAHA].

Vaidya-Jīvana: A short medical treatise composed by LOLIṀBA-RĀJA (*Lolamba-raja*) before A.D. 1600, in the manner of an ornate poem (kāvya). There is an erotic element in the poem, which is planned to be the author's address to his beloved (Murāsa or Ratna-mālā by name) concerning various ailments and their cures. The effort is both unique and interesting and it is successful as a medical work.

The author confesses that there is nothing original in this work (sva-kapola-kalpitam ihāsti na kiñchit, verse 6). He has compiled the formulae from earlier medical writers like Charaka, Suśruta and Vāgbhaṭa. In a little over 200 verses in elegant metres, he treats of fever, diarrhoea, grahaṇī (chronic diarrhoea), cough, asthma, rheumatism, eye-diseases, jaundice, women's ailments, tuberculosis, ulcers, urinary disorders, eczema, piles, acidity, heart-diseases, giddiness, dropsy, diseases of the teeth, ear and head. There is also a section on tonics and aphrodisiacs.

The prefatory verses enjoin that the physician must carefully determine the nature of the disease by standard methods, and consider the curability of the disease before beginning the treatment (v.8). There is a warning that the patient must reject the treatment offered by an ignorant physician (v.9). The author is convinced that medicines are unnecessary for the patient who is careful about food habits (pathya), and useless for one who is not (v.10). This verse is cleverly worded to convey a double meaning (pathye sati gadārtasya kim aushadha-nishevaṇam?); the second half of the verse repeats the words with a mark of elision between the first two words.

The work is frequently commented upon. Well-known is the commentary known as *Sukhānanda* (1910); other commentaries include *Dīpikā* (Harinātha-Gosvāmi, *Jagach-chandrikā* (Bhagīratha), *Vidyānanda-karī* (Prayāga-datta), and a gloss by Rudra-bhaṭṭa.

The work is also known as *Loliṁba-rājīyam [See* LOLIṀBA-RĀJĀ].

Vaidyaka-Śabda-Sindhu: An excellent modern medical dictionary in Sanskrit, compiled by Umesh-chandra Gupta (Calcutta, 1894), at the instance of Mahendralāl Sircār and with the support of Mahārājāh of Vizianagaram.

The work is voluminous and comprehensive. Terms of medical interest are arranged alphabetically, and brief descriptions of the drugs, diseases, recipes and preparations are given, along with relevant extracts from classical texts. The names of drugs are given not only in Sanskrit, but in Latin and in some modern Indian languages.

Vaṅgasena: Author of *Chikitsā-sāra-saṁgraha*, an encyclopaedic work on pathology and treatment (Calcutta 1884, ed. Nandakumār Goswāmi, 1889, and Jīvānanda-Vidyāsāgar, 1893). The oldest MSs of this work is dated A.D. 1276. The author's date is given as c. A.D. 1119 (before A.D. 1200, according to P.K. Goḍe).

Son of Gadādhara, he was born in Kaṇṭi-kāvāsa (village Kañjikā) in Bengal. He learnt medicine from his father (tātapādam gurum cha, prefatory verse), and compiled this immense work as "a collection of well-tried medical formulae from elders in the art of medicine" (vaidya-vṛddha-siddha-prayoga-nivaha, 1).

"Health is the necessary precondition for the four-fold human values (righteous living, wealth, pleasures and salvation); and diseases steal them away, and foil the very purpose of life. I shall here explain the pathology as well as treatment (*sa-nidāna-chikitsitam*) for these diseases" (prefatory verses 6 and 7).

The work consists of 104 sections (adhikāras), arranged on the model of *Mādhava-nidāna*; enumeration and description of diseases also follow the latter. But curative aspects and formulae are special features of this work. Each disease is considered under two heads: symptoms and causes (atha nidānam ... lakshaṇam āha), and treatment methods and drugs (atha chikisitam āha).

Despite the comprehensive character of the work, it is interesting that it is altogether silent about 'pulse-examination' (nāḍī-parīkshā), calcination of metals (although purification of quick-silver has been mentioned, 'rasa-parpaṭa', orbicular preparation with melted sulphur), and opium. His treatment of metals is all too cursory and meagre, apart from the reference to iron and steel while dealing with haemorrhoids.

The work is poetical, excepting in two sections (Nasyādhikāra and Saṁśodhana-saṁśamana- rasa-dravyādīnām vargādhi-kāra) where prose passages abound. The language throughout is elegant Sanskrit, and versification has not interfered with the scientific rigour or clarity.

The work has been consistently popular among physicians, especially in Bengal; and often selected portions of this work are committed to memory by students. The work describes diseases comprehensively and contains detailed accounts of treatments. The account given here of dietetics and pharmacology are excellent.

Vāryovida: An ancient medical authority quoted by Charaka *(CS, Sū. sth.*, ch. 12, vātakālakālīyam, 9 and ch.26, 8). He appears to have been a sage belonging to some royal family (rājarshi).

Participating in a conference concerning the wind (vāyu) both within the body and outside, the condition of its normalcy, the sources of its derangement (prakopanam), the methods of its reconstitution (upaśamāni), he gives a comprehensive account of the rôle of wind (vāyu) in the human constitution, in health and in disease. It supports the structure and function of the organism (tantra-yantra-dharah). It is distinguished by five operations: prāṇa, udāna, samāna, vyāna, apāna.

In its normalcy (akupitah), it motivates all behaviour (pravartakaś cheshṭānām), prompts and regulates mind (niyantā praṇetā cha manasah), activates all sense-organs (udyojakah sarvendriyāṇām), organizes all sensory function (sarvendriyārthānām abhivoḍhā), integrates all the constituents of the body (sarva-śarīra-dhātuvyūha-karah), unifies the bodily action (sandhāna-karah śarīrasya), stimulates speech (pravartako vachah), constitutes the very nature of touch and sound (prakṛitih sparśa-śabdayoh), functions as the root of auditory and cutaneous sensations (śrotra-sparśanayor yonih), fans the stomachic fire (samīraṇo-gneh), dries up and throws out the waste products (ksheptā bahir malānām), and facilitates the continuance of life (āyusho-nuvṛtti-pratyaya-bhūtah).

In its deranged condition, it produces various kinds of disturbances in the body, agitates the mind, generates grief, fear, confusion and anxiety, interferes with the fivefold functions (prāṇa, apāna etc.), and cuts down happiness and life.

He winds up the discussion with an eloquent eulogy on wind as the very godhead (vāyur eva bhagavān iti), which provokes another sage Marīchi to inquire what use is all this knowledge for a physician. Marīchi reminds Vāryovida that the conference is interested only in matters of medicine (bhishag-vidyām adhikṛtya yam kathā prāvartata iti). Vāryovida retorts that without a theoretical understanding of the normal and abnormal conditions of the wind, a physician would not be able to handle the wind to the best advantage of the patient, and would not know how to restore the deranged wind to its normalcy [*See* MARĪCHI].

He agrees generally with the views of Baḍīsa as regards the derangement and restoration of the wind in the body [*See* BAḌĪŚA].

There is an interesting viewpoint that is ascribed to Vāryovida (*CS, Sū. sth.*, ch.25,12-13). He rejects the all-important role of mind in the causation of diseases [*See* ŚARALOMA]. He accepts the involvement of mind in bodily ailments, but bodily ailments cannot occur without direct physiological causes, the three *doshas* (narte śarīrāc chārīra-rogāh). Further, he argues, mind cannot function independent of the body (na manasah sthitih). Chkp. adds ṛte śarīrād iti yojyam, and explains that the mind being saturated with rajas and tamas will always be within the physiological context. Śivadāsasena takes this statement to mean that mind is not involved even in the production of the body; mind, he suggests, emerges only after the body gets formed. He concedes, however, that mind is the chief source of mental diseases (mānasa-rogeshu eva manasah kāraṇatvam).

He held that tastes (rasa) are six in number: heavy (guru), light (laghu), cool (śīta), hot (ushṇa), unctuous (snigdha), and dry, coarse or astringent (rūksha). These differences in qualities (guṇa-bhedah), and in action (karma-bhedah) are due to the different tastes (rasa-kṛta eva) (cf. Chkp. on *CS*, 1,26,8). Ātreya agrees that tastes are six only, but enumerates them as sweet (madhura), sour (amla), saltish (lavaṇa), acrid (kaṭu), bitter (tikta), and astringent (kashāya) (*CS*, 1,26,9).

Vijaya-rakshita: He is the author of *Madhukośa* (along with Śrīkaṇṭha-Datta), a commentary on *MN*, a 13th century work.

His commentary closes abruptly at the end of section 32 (on calculus, *aśmarī*), and it is continued and completed by his student, Śrīkaṇṭha-Datta.

The prefatory verse (5) remembers the earlier medical authorities: Bhaṭṭāra (-Harichandra?), Jaijjaṭa, Gadādhara, Vāpya-Chandra, Chkp, Bakula, Īśvara-Sena, Bhoja, Iśāna, Kārtika, Śukra, Sudhīra, Maitreya and Mādhava; and claims to have examined all other related disciplines (tantrāntarāṇy api vilokya). The commentary promises to supply during the course of the commentary diagnostic material that will be useful, but left unsaid by the author Mādhava (upayuktam ihānuktam nidānam Mādhavena yat; grantha-vyākhyā-prasaṅgena mayā tadapi likhyate). The promise is amply fulfilled [*See* MADHU-

KOSHA].

Vīrasiṁhāvaloka: A work written by, or for, a Rajput prince VĪRASIṀHA (son of Tomāra-deva-varman) who lived around 1380, it seeks to press astrological details for the aetiology and treatment of diseases. It is one of the early works that bring astrology within the field of medicine, the earliest being *AHr*. It claims that the royal author has prepared this work for the welfare of the world (viśvopakāra), having churned the milky oceans of astrology, Vedic lore (āgama), dharma-śāstra, tantra (nigama) and medicine (āyurveda).

Veterinary science: Care of domesticated animals has been a continuous preoccupation with Indian physicians, all through the country's history, both in the villages and in the royal courts. The pastoral economy during the Vedic times, and earlier in the Indus Valley civilization, made this concern relevant to social life. Horses, elephants, cattle, camels and buffaloes have been harnessed to human use, and have been regarded as valuable possessions.

And thus a fairly extensive literature grew up concerning the animals, their classification, identification of breed, nature, rearing, training, management, anatomy, diseases and treatment. Unfortunately much of this literature is lost. But the available portions and references indicate the comprehensive character of many of these works.

A branch of Indian medicine developed along the veterinary direction, principally dealing with the care and cure of horses, *(hayāyurveda)*, elephants (gajāyurveda), and cattle (*gav āyurveda*). ŚĀLIHOTRA, PĀLAKĀPYA and SAHADEVA are prominent authors of standard texts on horses, elephants and cattle respectively. There is a book on hawks also (*Śyainika-śāstra*) by RUDRADEVA of Kumaon. It may be recalled that hawks were not only pets in royal households, but were used for communication, sports and entertainment.

The general orientation of veterinary science in India followed in the main the basic position of Āyurveda: the pañcha-bhūta theory, the tri-dosha doctrine, and the adequacy of herbal medicine. Surgical operations also were frequently conducted on animals and special instruments were designed for this purpose. Care of the sick animals was considered, and numerous prescriptions have been given in this regard. There were hospitals specially meant for animals as can be gleaned from the edicts of emperor Aśoka. The villages had peripatetic cattle-physicians (go-vaidyas), and kings and chieftains patronized specialists in diagnosing and treating the diseases of horses and elephants. *Hārīta-saṁhitā* (3,2) speaks of physicians who treated not only human beings but also animals (like deer, snakes and rodents).

The diseases of horses and their treatment constituted an early concern. Śālihotra, Garga and Nakula are celebrated authors on the subject. Several *purāṇas* (e.g. *Agni-*, 281, *Gāruḍa-*, 197 and 207, and *Matsya-*, 189 and 191) deal with this topic, and give extracts from standard texts like *Śālihotra*. So does *Nīti-sāra* of Śukra. Nakula, a Pāṇḍava hero in *Mahābhārata*, was reputed to be an authority on horses; *Aśva-chikitsā* in his name has come down to us (ed. Umesh Chandra Gupta, *Bibl. Indica*, 1887).

Other works include Bhoja's *Śālihotra* (11th century, *Munich Catal.*, Jolly), Dīpaṁkara's *Aśva-vaidyaka*, Jayadatta-sūri's work of the same name (1500 *Bibl. Indica*, 1887, ed. by U.C. Gupta; also ed. Jībānanda Vidyāsāgar), Gaṇa's *Aśvāyurveda*, Sārṅgadhara's *Vāji-chikitsā*, and Indusena's *Śālihotra-sāra-saṁgraha* (1812). There are several references to other works on the subject, which however are no longer available (like *Haya-līlāvati*, *Revottara* and *Aśva-śāstra*, mentioned by the commentator Mallinātha on the Sanskrit poem *Śiśupālavadha*, 5,60). Simha-datta's voluminous work on horses (described as *aśva-śāstra-samudram*) (No. 13318 of GOML, 38) has also been lost.

PĀLAKAPYA's work deals comprehensively with the diseases and treatment of elephants (ed. Anandāśrama Series, Poona). The subject was a favourite one during the Mughal rule, and the traveller al-Berūni quotes from a work of this kind. Other works on the same subject include *Mātaṅga-līla* and *Gaja-chikitsā*. Kauṭilya's *Arthaśāstra* and Kāmaṇḍaka's *Nīti-sāra* deal with the subject. There is an elaborate account of it also in *Agni-purāṇa* (289-91).

SAHADEVA's *Gavāyurveda* is no longer available, but the tradition of cattle-treatment (go-vaidya) that it contained became widespread in the country. *Agni-purāṇa* deals with the subject in an elaborate manner. *Parāśara-saṁhitā* contains references to cattle-care and cattle-physicians.

Vopadeva: He was a prolific writer who lived around A.D. 1300. Among his works two are medical in content: (1) *Vaidya-śata-ślokī* (containing a hundred recipes that contribute to health) and (2) *Siddha-mantra prakāśa*, a commentary on his father' *Siddha-mantra* (a work in 170 verses).

Son of the physician Keśava of Vidarbha (Berar) he migrated to Devagiri (Aurangabad district, Maharashtra). He was patronized by HEMĀDRI, who was minister to the Yādava Kings of Devagiri, Mahādeva (1260-1271) and Rāmachandra-Deva (1271-1309). He studied under the reputed physicians, Dineśa and Bhāskara.

His father Keśava-bhishak composed *Siddha-mantra* which was a sort of medical glossary as well as *materia medica*. Vopadeva's *Prakāśa* on it is elaborate and gives information about how to prepare and administer medicines like pills and powders (Madras, 1860).

Vṛnda (Vṛnda-Kuṇḍa): Author of *Siddha-yoga*, a standard medical manual, which influenced Chakrapāṇi-Datta. The work frequently mentions diseases which were prevalent in Western India; it is therefore suggested that he hailed from that part of the country. Nothing is known about him, except that he was a devotee of Śiva, Chaṇḍī and Gaṇeśa (who figure in the initial verse). He, in humility, describes himself as "dull-witted" (Vṛndena manda-matinā) and claims that he wrote this work which 'determines the diseases' (gada-viniśchaya), for his own spiritual welfare (ātma-hitārthinā).

He is assigned to the 9th century A.D. , as Chkp has used many of his formulae [*See* SIDDHA-YOGA].

Y

Yoga-ratnākara: An anonymous and extensive compilation of medical formulae, padded with valuable information concerning health, hygiene, eight-fold examination of the patient (aṣṭha-sthāna-parīkshā), seasonal requirements, beneficient food articles and habits, weights and measures, pharmacy, metallurgical procedures, toxicology, and five-fold treatment procedures (pañcha-karma). Anatomy and surgery are excluded from its scope.

A MSS of this work, dated 1746, is available. But when precisely this work was composed is not known. It must be later than *BP*, for new preparations from *Chopachīnī* are given here. But syphilis (phiraṅga) mentioned in *BP* is not to be found here.

The work appears to be indebted to *Bṛhad-yoga-Taraṅgiṇī,* both in its content and style.

The work was published in the Ānandāśrama Sanskrit Series, Pune in 1889. Part I of this work was published in Mysore in 1899 (Govt. Oriental Library with annotations in Kannada and Telugu). Part II, as yet unpublished, deals with disease categories along with their diagnostic details and treatment procedures, toxicology, rejuvenation and aphrodisiacs.

The significance of this compendium consists in the unprecedented emphasis on the curative value of 'proper food, drink and conduct' (Pathya) in various diseases as well as specific prescriptions in this regard. While the rest of the work is largely a mere compilation, the claim in this context is that a special effort was made to ascertain the *pathya* aspect in earlier medical works (ālokya vaidya-tantrād esha nibadhyate; vyādhitānām chikitsātham pathyāpthya-viniśchayah). According to the compiler, the three essential ingredients of successful treatment are diagnosis (nidāna), medicine (aushadha) and pathya; he therefore suggests that the physician must consider them carefully (triṇi yatnena chintayet).

Another interesting detail found here is the account of tobacco (tamākhu), which is said to cure cough, asthma, flatulence, troubles of the teeth, and excesses of kapha and vāta, but to produce giddiness, vomiting, purging and optical ailments (section 557).

There is an elaborate account of 'night life' *(rātri-charyā)* dealing principally with healthy sex activities (vv. 409-441). This is a theme that is usually not covered in earlier medical works. Useful properties of several grains, vegetables, fruits and different kinds of meat as articles of food are listed (vv. 481-600). Recipes (kṛtānna) are also indicated.

Judging from the recipes given, the compiler appears to hail from Mahārāshtra, from where the MSS was also recovered and where the work is popular. (Ānandāśrama Sanskrit Series, 1889).

Yoga-Śataka: Pelliot's archaeological expedition in the Kucha region (Central Asia) discovered this text in Sanskrit along with Kuchaen translation.

Ascribed to the great Nāgārjuna (in Tibetan Klu-grub), the text is extant in its Tibetan version *(Sbyor-ba brgva-pa),* prepared by Jetakarṇa Buddha-śrī-jñana and Ñi-ma rgyal-mtshan, and included in the Bstan-hgyur (Tanjūr) division of the Tibetan Buddhist canon. There is extant in Sanskrit another work with the same title, ascribed to Vararuchi, which bears a close resemblance with the Tibetan work (cf. Bhagwan Dash: *Tibetan Medicine, with special reference to Yoga-Śataka,* Library of Tibetan Works and Archives, Dharamsala, 1976).

The Tibetan work consists of 125 verses, with two additional verses by the translators. The first two verses appear to be by them. Verse 4 describes the formulae as ambrosia and describes the value of accurate examination of the disease, its causation, and signs. The next verse describes the 'eight organs' of Āyurveda, including 'Pañchakarma' as the eighth and omitting the usual vājikaraṇa from the list.

The work purports to give one hundred medicinal formulae "which are praised by expert physicians" (beginning with verse 6), arranged in the standard division into general physical ailments (kāya-chikitsā), diseases of head and neck (śālākya), surgical condition (śalya), toxicology (agada), psychiatry (bhūtavidyā), paediatrics (śiśu-roga-śamana), and rejuvenation (rasāyana), There are further sections (uttara) dealing with the five specialized therapies (pañcha-karma) (v.v. 98-102), useful single drugs (26 in number) for common ailments (v. 103), and treatment for the doshas (v.v. 106-121).

The work ends with an admonition that the physician should comprehend both what is expressly stated in the book and what is left unsaid; and that he should above all understand the disease itself before he attempts to cure, and that he must decide upon the course of treatment in his own wisdom (v. 123).

The work in the canonical collection has been supplied by an annotation (chen) by the celebrated scholiast Bu-ston Rin-po-che (1299-1364)

There are several texts of *Yoga-Śataka* in Sanskrit (not the same as the above, but similar to it) discovered in Nepal, Ceylon and different parts of India. Prescriptions of *Yoga-Śataka* were popular in Ceylon.

Appendix

Selections bearing on the History of Indian Medicine

I. THE AŚVINS AS PHYSICIANS OF GODS AND MEN

RV, 5, 73,—

Come, O Aśvins who partake of a share in many sacrificial offerings, come whether you are close at hand or far off, or in different places.(1).

I invite the two of you, who encourage those that approach you, who are great achievers, who are the most adored, and who never fail.(2)

You have arrested one of the wheels of your chariot in order to increase the glory of the Sun; and with the other wheel, you traverse the spheres to regulate (the activities of days and nights.(3)

Leaders that you are, Atri (our ancestor) acknowledged with gratitude your help when he found relief from the intense 'heat' that he was suffering from.(6)

O Aśvins, rightly did the sages of yore praise you as bestowers of happiness (health). We welcome you to come in our midst and bestow (on us) happiness.(9)

RV, 5, 74,—

Denizens of the higher realms and affluent in mental powers, O ye Aśvins, descend upon the earth and listen to our prayers. The son of Atri approaches you with prayers so that you may shower benefits on us.(1)

O Aśvins, you have stripped the old sage Chyavana of his worn out form like a dilapidated armour; you have made him young again, and desired by women.(5)

[Note: The legend of Chyavana's rejuvenation is given in Śatapatha-brāhmaṇa, (4.1.5): Śaryāti, the King, was angered by his frolicksome daughter, Sukanyā, whom he gave away in marriage to an old sage, Chyavana. When this young girl was residing in Chyavana's hermitage, the Aśvins approached her and asked her to marry them. The girl refused to accede to their desire, and expressed her resolve to live with her old husband. Later, the Aśvins, requested by her, suggested that the sage should bathe in a particular pond; and when he did so youth was restored to him. *cf.* also RV,1,117,13; 1,118,6; 5,74,5; 7,71,5 and 10,39,4. *cf.* also RV, 1,112,15 where Kali was similarly rejuvenated.]

Here is your devotee! May we ever be under your care, and prosperous. Listen to my prayer, and come to me with your numerous benefits and succour.(6)

Your chariot which is the swiftest of chariots, which frightens the foes and which is adored by the humans, may that chariot draw near us, well-disposed towards us.(8)

RV, 5, 75,—

Aśvins who are masters of the mystic lore, heed to my words of welcome! I adorn with words of praise your excellent chariot, beloved of men, bestower of benefits and carrier of comforts.(1)

[Note: 1. The chariot in which the Aśvins travel is said to have three wheels, representing residence and travel in the three spheres, *viz.,* earth, mid-region and the heavens. *cf.* RV,5,76,4.

The chariot is thus described as 'tridhātu', constituted of three elements (RV,8,39,9). Sāyaṇa explains that the three elements refer to earth (prithvi) (viz., food), water (āp) and fire (tejas). Elsewhere the expression is made to signify the three guṇas, viz. sattva, rajas, and tamas (RV,8,47,10), the three colours, viz., white, black and red (RV,5,43,13), or three vital currents, viz., prāṇa, apāna and vyāna (RV,3,26,7).]

[Note: 2. Aśvins are addressed here as 'masters of the mystic lore' (mādhvī), which expression is explained by the commentators (Sāyaṇa and Skandasvāmin) as referring to the following legend included in Vājasaneya-brāhmaṇa. Indra taught the sage Dadhīchi (Dadhyañch) son of Ātharvaṇa, the mystic doctrine of Brahman known as 'Madhu', but warned him against teaching it to others on pain of losing his head. The Aśvins approached the sage for learning this same doctrine. When the sage refused to teach them and told them why, the Aśvins offered to provide him with another head, in case he lost his. Then the sage taught them. When his head fell off, the Aśvins brought a horse's head and fixed it on his shoulders. *cf.* also RV,1,119,9.].

The dawn has arrived. The season's fire has settled on the altar and is blazing forth. O Aśvins, who bestow wealth and vanquish the enemies, your immortal chariot is in readiness to travel. Come, and listen to my prayers.(9).

RV, 5, 76,—

O Aśvins, spoil not the perfect (rite)! Come, and we will adore you here. Arrive at dawn and bring us your protections against unhappiness, and bestow prosperity on the performer of the rite.(2)

May we be joined with the Aśvins, equipped with their protection, which secures happiness to us and enables us to lead a good life. O immortal Aśvins, shower on us wealth, progeny and other good things in life.(5)

RV, 5, 77,—

Your splendid chariot, covered with gold and delightful like honey, exudes (health-giving) liquids, and is heading towards us, fast as wind and quick like thought, to our succour, O ye Aśvins.(3)

[**Note:** See below Note on RV,1,119,1]

RV, 5, 78,—

O Aśvins, liberate from the wooden box the frightened and imploring sage, Saptavadhrī, with your wondrous skill.(6)

[**Note:** The legend of the sage is given in the commentary. The brothers of this sage became jealous of him, and attempted to prevent his nightly intercourse with his beautiful wife so that he may not beget children. They imprisoned him every night in a big box made of wood, and belaboured him severely during the day. The unhappy sage, who also became ill and emaciated, implored the aid of the Aśvins. They promptly arrived, freed him from his captivity and restored his health. The sage could thus unite with his wife and beget a child. *cf* verses 7, 8 and 9, where prayers are addressed to the Aśvins for safe delivery.]

RV,1,116,—

O Aśvins who are leaders of men on the path of good, you bestowed sharp and wide intelligence to Kakshīvat of the Pajra family. You made your horses exude the invigorating drink by their very hooves, and filled a hundred pots.(7)

[**Note:** The sage Kakshīvat, thirty-third in the line of the Āngira-sages, became mentally deficient, owing to an illness. The Aśvins cured him, probably by a rasāyana formula. The sage then became renowned for his brilliant mind (puraṁdhī). *cf.* also 1,117,6.]

You cured, with a cold infusion (hima), the intense heat (gharma) of Atri; you nourished him with food, and extricated him safely from the dark cavern into which the demons had driven him.(8)

[**Note:** The legend given by the commentators narrates that a group of demons kidnapped the sage and held him in captivity. They also set fire to him. When he implored the Aśvins to come to his aid, they poured water on the fire, and freed him from his confinement. But this seems to be a symbolic narration of the sage being cured of his high fever, burning sensations, loss of appetite, and depression. It is usual in the Vedic hymns for diseases to be referred to as demons.

Significant also is the employment of the expression 'hima' in the verse, which is obviously a medicinal preparation of cold water. Skandasvāmin interprets the word to mean 'rain-water' (vṛshṭiudaka) *cf.* also RV, 1,118,7; 5,78,4-6; 7,70,5; 8,62,3, etc; 10,39,9.]

O disapprovers of falsehood, you brought the well to the thirsty sage Gotama, and upturned it so that he may drink his fill.(9)

[**Note:** Gotama was travelling in a desert, and was tormented by excessive thirst. He prayed to the Aśvins, who helped him. *cf.* RV, 1,85,11, where this feat is ascribed to the Maruts. But the allegory suggests the relief that the sage obtained from a disease characterized by abnormal thirst. The well that the Aśvins brought to the sage is intriguingly described in the verse as 'bottom turned upwards'. Does it refer to a treatment?]

Human leaders that you are, you came to know how Vandana was hidden (in a well) in an unfrequented region, like a treasure; and you recovered him. This courageous deed of yours is truly praiseworthy, adorable, and desired by us.(11)

[**Note:** Vandana, the sage, was dragged by the demons to a deserted jungle, and pushed into a well. The verse speaks of the well being recognized by the passersby *(darśatāt),* who however were unable to come to the aid of the unfortunate sage. The Aśvins pulled him out. Even here, the reference is to a grave illness which troubled the sage, and which was cured by the Aśvins. Elsewhere (RV,1,119,7), there is reference to the same sage who is here described as emaciated, and whom the Aśvins rendered young and long-lived. Another sage Rebha, was in a similar predicament, (viz., 'pushed into a well'), and the Aśvins are said to have saved him (RV, 1,112,5). *cf.* also RV 1,112,5; 1,119,6; 1,118,6; 10,39,8.]

O Aśvins, who protect the folk and fulfil the desires of people, the princes Vadhrimatī sought your aid, and you gave her splendid arms.(13)

[**Note:** According to the commentator Skandasvāmin, Vadhrimatī was a warrior-princess, who lost her arms in a battle and the Aśvins provided her with artificial limbs made of gold plates (hiraṇya-hasta). Sāyaṇa, however, interprets the word Vadhrimati to mean 'one who had an impotent husband (vadhri); the Aśvins cured him of this defect, and eventually he became the father of a male child named Hiraṇya-hasta. *cf.* also RV, 1,117,24; 6,62,7; 10,39,7.]

O disapprovers of falsehood, you saved the life of a sparrow (vartikā) from the clutches of a wolf (vṛka). You gave sight to the blind poet who implored your help. Such is your competence and benefaction to many.(14)

[**Note:** *cf.* also RV, 1,117,16; 1,118,8; 10,39,13.]

You provided even in the darkness of a night iron legs to Viśpalā, the lady of the prince Khela, when her legs were severed, like the wings of a bird, in the course of a battle; she could walk and carry the treasure to safety.(15)

[**Note:** The legend is that the prince Khela was engaged in a war with his enemies, the bone of contention being some treasure. His wife Viśpalā, was also fighting on the battlefield; the enemy attacked her and cut off her legs, when it was dark. The prince's priest Agastya invoked the assistance of the Aśvins, who immediately arrived and provided her with artificial limbs made of iron. She was made fit enough to walk instantly, *cf.* also 1,117,11; 1,118,8; 10,39,8.]

When Ṛjrāśva was cursed by his father to become blind, for cutting up a hundred sheep to feed his wolf, you physicians came to his help and gave him sight.(16)

[**Note:** Ṛjrāśva was the profligate son of King Vṛshāgira. This young man had a pet wolf (which was actually the transformation of the mount of the Aśvins). To feed it, the prince was in the habit of collecting sheep belonging to his people. The king was annoyed at this outrage against his people, and caused his son to become blind. The Aśvins, however, took pity on him and repaired his eyes. *cf.* also RV, 1,117,17 and 1,120,6.

It is significant that the Aśvins are described here as 'physicians' (bhishajau). *cf.* also Aitareya-brāhmaṇa, 1,18; Taittirīyāsamhitā 2,3,11.]

O disapprovers of falsehood and the ever-young ones, you easily carried to safety the sage Jāhusa, who was surrounded by deadly foes (viz., who was besieged by numerous diseases); and he was placed in a place inaccessible to enemies (viz., he was made healthy and resistant to diseases).(20)

O Aśvins, having praised your skill (in healing), may I desire to live well and long, prosperous and healthy (lit., with my eyesight intact) and enter into old age as one enters his own home. (25)

RV, 1, 117,—

O charming ones, you extricated the sage Vandana who had been hidden in the well, who was like one who was stretched upon the ground, like the sun who was hidden in the night, but who was lustrous like some splendid ornament.(5)

[**Note:** 'Hidden in the well' suggests being old and worn out (*cf.* 1,119,7) or in a state of deep depression, probably symptomatic of a mental illness. There was also a catatonic involvement, suggested by being stretched on the ground. The absence of any physical disease is suggested by the similes of the sun and the lustrous ornament. *cf.* also Note on RV, 1,116,11.]

O leaders of men, the two of you restored to Viśvaka (son of Kṛshṇa) his lost son, Vishṇvāpu, and bestowed on the old maid Ghoshā, languishing in her father's house, a husband. (7)

[**Note:** 1. Viśvaka's son was gravely ill and was given up for lost; the Aśvins were able to cure the boy. One commentary suggests that the son had gone away and that the Aśvins brought him back. Skandasvāmin, however, explains that the boy was dead, and that the Aśvins resuscitated him. *cf.* RV, 1,116,23; 10,65,12.]

[**Note:** 2. Ghoshā, the learned daughter of the sage Kakshīvat, became afflicted by an incurable skin disease (kushṭa), and was therefore abandoned by her husband. She had to return to her father's house, and languish there without a hope of cure or of normal family life. The Aśvins, however, cured her, and made her husband accept her again. *cf.* also RV 10,39, 3 and 6; 10,4,5. Two hymns in RV (10,39 and 40) are ascribed to her.]

O Aśvins, you bestowed on the leper sage Śyāva a charming bride, on the floundering Kaṇva eyesight, and on Nārshada the faculty of hearing. Praiseworthy indeed are your deeds.(8)

[**Note:** 1. The Śyāva, the eldest son of the sage Ghora, who was the son of Agni was afflicted by a serious skin disease (leprosy) which had turned his skin dark and hideous. His thighs had withered, and his head had become deformed. The Aśvins corrected these conditions, eliminated the source of the disease, and restored the young man to health, so that he could marry. This is the explanation of Skandasvāmin. *cf.* also RV,1,117,24.]

[**Note:** 2. The sage Kaṇva had lost his eyesight, and was unable to move about. The Aśvins restored his eye-sight (taijasam chakshur indriyam) (Sāyaṇa and Skandasvāmin).]

[**Note:** 3. The son of Nṛshada, a sage, was hard of hearing. The *asuras,* to test his supernatural powers, confined him in a dark cell in the night with a promise that he would be set free if he could tell when it dawned. The Aśvins in the meantime came to him and corrected his auditory defect. He could hear the strains of music when the

Aśvins played on Vīṇā at dawn, and could thus secure his freedom. Skandasvāmin gives the name of this boy as Kaṇva.]

O removers of distress, your devotee Tugra was anxious about his son who was being tossed about in an agitated ocean. You saved this boy with your speedy boats and swift horses. The grateful father had reason to praise you afresh.(14)

[**Note:** The 'agitated ocean' refers to serious illness; 'the boats and horses' refer to treatment-methods and drugs. See below Note on RV,1,119,4.]

O the praise-worthy Aśvins, the care bestowed on us by the two of you has made us happy. You have rendered the diseased folk (srāmam) healthy (sam riṇītah). It is therefore that the clever Ghosā has addressed her prayers to you, the wish-fulfillers.(19)

[**Note:** Ghoshā the learned lady (brahmavādinī) was troubled by an ailment, and sought the help of the Aśvins to cure her (rogopaśamanārtham) (Sāyaṇa).]

O worthy ones to behold (dasra), you made Śayu's old, milkless, and barren cow young and full of milk. You also made by your expert device Purumitra's daughter a wife to Vimada.(20)

[**Note:** Purumitra's daughter also was barren, like Śayu's cow. The Aśvins effected a cure for this condition.]

O generous and compassionate leaders of men, you gave golden arms to Vadhrimatī, and you rendered whole and alive the body of Śyāva, which was cut into three bits. (24)

[**Note:** 1.See above Note on RV 1,116,13.]

[**Note** 2. The sage Syava was afflicted by leprosy (kushṭhita), and his body was thus deformed and mutilated. The Aśvins treated him and made him wholesome. Skandasvāmin suggests that they operated on his body at three places, or in three different ways (tribhih prakāraih), as a part of treatment. See also above Note on RV,1,117,8.]

RV, 1, 118,—

Come to us in your excellent chariot, which has three seats and three wheels, and which is triangular in shape. Fill our cows with milk and our horses with energy, and make us prosperous.(2)

[**Note:** The verse describes the desirability of the medical care. The Aśvins are welcome to the mortals who need to be healthy and wealthy. But the three-fold details are obscure. The 'seat' (vandhura) is the place where the driver sits. Sāyaṇa explains that this seat is constructed on three columns (?). The idea of three wheels, however, has been explained as referring to three dhātus (see above Note 1 on RV 5,75,1).

It may be that the three 'seats' (or columns) refer to the three *guṇas* (sattva, rajas and tamas), the three 'wheels' to the three dhātus (vāta, pitta and śleshman), and the triangular shape to the three treatment procedures (kāyachikitsā, śalya and rasāyana).]

Come, O charmers, come in your splendid chariot and listen to the praises of this devotee. Truly have the sages of yore described the two of you as most prompt in relieving the misery of those that seek you.(3)

O charmers, who also shower benefits on people, you helped with your valiant deeds Vandana and Rebha (who had 'fallen into the well', viz., become dejected), the son of Tugra (Bhujyu, who was being tossed about in the stormy sea, *viz.*, who was anxious and agitated), and Chyavana (who had become old and infirm).(6)

[**Note:** The verse refers to three kinds of deeds that the Aśvins are celebrated for: raising up people who are hidden in the well, bringing back to safety those who are caught in the violent sea, and restoring youth. The three probably refer to the therapeutics (for milder ailments), surgery (for more serious ailments), and rasāyana (for rejuvenation).]

O Aśvins, you relieved Atri of the intense heat that he was suffering from, you also gave him food that nourished and delighted him, you gave bright vision to Kanva who was blinded by a cover (cataract?).(7)

O leaders of men and well-born ones, come to us in your excellent chariot, come to our succour, and bring us prosperity, well pleased with our words of welcome.(10)

RV, 1, 119,—

We, who need nourishment, O Aśvins, invoke your splendid chariot, which is filled with many miracles, swift like thought, drawn by fast-moving steed, adorned by many banners, rich in water, abundant in food, and productive of happiness.(1)

[**Note:** The Aśvin's chariot signifies the therapeutics that they were famous for. The cure effected by them was miraculous; the recovery was fast and permanent. They administered their medicine in water, and along with food. They made the patient wholesome and happy. *cf.* RV 1,120,10, where their chariot is described as 'without horses' (anaśvam).

There are diverse descriptions of their chariot. It is entirely made of gold (RV 1, 1,80,1; 4,44,4;8,5,29; 8,22,8). It is drawn by asses (rāsabha. RV, 1,34,9; 1,116,2 also Nirukta, 2,28); by horses (1,117,2); by birds (6,63,6); by swans (4,45,4); by eagle (garuda), (1,18,4); by horses in the shape of falcons (8,5,7). The Aśvins are never described as riders of horses, although the expression 'Aśvin' suggests their possession of horses (aśva).

The daughter of the sun (Sūryā) is said to travel with them in their chariot, which is fast like the thought (manojava) and which is protected in all ways (śtotih), and which travels across the worlds to the one who invokes them (RV, 7,68,3). Drawn by powerful steed, the golden chariot of the Aśvins is said to block up heaven and earth (rodasī), and come to men for their succour, following the track of waters (7,69,1). The chariot is renowned among the five orders of beings (pañcha-bhuma) (7,69,2). It contributes to our purification (śam) and happiness (yoh) (7,69,5).]

You have recovered by your own devices Bhujyu, who was lost, and returned him from afar to his father's home. You have also saved from great distress the King Divodāsa.(4)

[**Note:** *cf.* also 1,117,14. The legend given by Sāyaṇa is as follows. Bhujyu was the son of Tugra, a King. The enemies of the King had stationed themselves in a distant island and were causing him trouble. The King sent his son Bhujyu with an army to drive them away. But the boat in which Bhujyu was travelling to the island broke in mid-sea; and Bhujyu was helpless. He implored the Aśvins to come to his aid. They hurried to him with their own boats and horses and brought him back to land in safety.

But the verse is obviously allegorical. The Aśvins are invoked only in cases of disease, injury and anxiety due to disease. Bhujyu is described as being 'lost' (gatam), and there is no mention of sea in the verse; and it would be absurd to employ horses to recover a drowning man in the sea. The expression 'by your own devices' (sva-yuktibhih) does not suggest 'by your own horses and boats'. Bhujyu was ill, and gravely so. He had gone so far away from the world of living, that his recovery due to the treatment that the Aśvins administered became celebrated.

References to Bhujyu's distress and the Aśvins' help are frequent in RV. *cf.* also 8,5,22; 10,39,4; 10,47,7; 10,65,12 etc. Interesting is the reference (7,68,7) that Bhujyu was brought to distress by those who seemed friendly to him (sakhāyah) but in reality wished him ill (durevāsah). Is there a suggestion here that excessive indulgence in luxury can cause distress?

cf. RV 1,182,5-7, where the Aśvins are said to have fashioned a 'boat' which was 'alive' (ātmanvantam) and 'equipped with wings' (pakshiṇam) for Bhujyu (son of Tugṛa) to save him from the dark and deep sea. Four of such 'boats' were sent to him, with the help of which Bhujyu was able to come up, even as birds fly up in the air with the help of their wings.]

O charmers, skilled as you are, you restored youth to Vandana who was old and worn out (even as a wheelwright repairs) an old cart. You also delivered that sage from the womb of his mother (kshetrāt). May (such) beneficient acts of yours protect those who seek you (vidhate).(7)

[**Note:** Vandana's rejuvenation has already been mentioned. The sage who was delivered by the Aśvins is said to be Vāmadeva (Sāyaṇa). This is a case of difficult labour in which the Aśvins exhibited their skill.]

RV, 1, 120,—

O Aśvins, you have bestowed on people great (benefits) (mahah). You have rid people of great (distress) (niratatam satam). You afford us abode. Become our saviours, and guard from the powerful wolf (vṛka, viz., death).(7)

RV, 8, 73,—

O Aśvins, you freed Atri from the heat by cold (infusion) (hima). May your protection be close at hand.(3)

The Aśvins, are welcome in times of distress (yāmahūtamā). I should secure intimate relation with them. May the protection of the two of you be close at hand.(5)

RV, 8, 89,—

The charming Aśvins, physicians (bhishajā) that you are, you bring happiness to people (mayobhuvā). You were praised by Daksha. Now Viśvaka invokes you for the sake of his son! Do not spurn our friendship, and unyoke your chariot when you come to us (viz., abide with us). (1)

RV, 8, 22,—

O Aśvins, come to us with the same protections quick and sure, that you offered to Paktha, Adhrigu and Babhru; come and heal the sick (bhishajyatam yad āturam).(10)

The Aśvins are the masters of the waters (śubhapati), and they enter where distress is (rudra-vartini). I invoke them at dawn and during the rest of the day. O healers (rudrau), who are rich in nourishing food (vājinīvasū) leave us not at the mercy of the enemy.(14)

[**Note:** The Aśvins are addressed as the Rudras (lit., 'terrible ones' or 'shouting ones'), but the word also signifies 'those who drive away distress'). Rudra is also associated with the art of healing; he is called 'the best among physicians' (bhishaktama). *cf.*, RV, 2,33,4. The enemy referred to in the above verse is obviously disease.]

Abide close to us, with your numerous and quick protections, for our safety (avase), O the rainers of benefits, who are fast like thought, who protect the devoted and subdue the arrogant.(16)

May we obtain from you, O Aśvins, strength (suvīryam), happiness (sushṭhu), and what is desired by all (vāryam), and what is not struck down! May we obtain all the benefits (vāmāni, good things in life), when you, rich in nourishing food (vājinīvasū) come to us.(18)

RV, 10,39,—

O Aśvins, inspire our truthful songs! Fulfil our intentions and acts (dhiyah)! Enliven (udīrayantam) our many-dimensioned intellects (puraṁdhīh)! We need all these. And bestow on us the wealth that we cherish. Establish us thus amidst the prosperous, like the delightful Soma.(2)

O Aśvins, you have helped the old maid that languished in her father's home without the prospect of marriage; you have also helped the lowly (apamasya, i.e., bedridden), the poor of vision (andhasya), and emaciated (kṛśasya). You are truly the healers of the distressed (bhishajā rutasya).(3)

O Aśvins, the two of you are physicians that bestow great benefits (bhishajā mayobhuvā)! Therefore do we sing your ancient exploits in this direction (purāṇā vīrya) in the world, for our well-being (avase).(5)

I (Ghoshā) implore you O Aśvins, and pay heed to my words! Give me comfort (śikshatam) even as the parents afford to their child. Save me from the imminent curse before it strikes me and renders me helpless (anāpih), unconscious (ajña), despondent (asajātyā), and shorn of wit (amatih).(6).

[**Note:** Sāyaṇa takes the word śikshatam to mean wealth (dhanam). He interprets anāpih as devoid of relatives, ajña as devoid of gratitude, asajātyā as devoid of faith, and amatih as devoid of wisdom, and all these as attributes of the curse.]

You lent your chariot for Śundhyu, the daughter of Purumitra, to be carried to the residence of her husband Vimada. You were invoked by Vadhrimatī of brilliant mind, and you came to her succour.(7)

[**Note:** 1. Vimada was the sage who gave eight hymns in RV (10,20-27). When he married the daughter of Purumitra, he wanted to take her home in great style. The Aśvins arrived and conducted the bride and bride-groom in their own chariot to the latter's home (Sāyaṇa). But the reference here is probably to some ailment of the girl which prevented her from being accepted by her husband.]

[**Note:** 2. About Vadhrimatī, *cf.*, Note above on RV 1,116,13. The expression 'su-shutim chakratuh' has been explained by Sāyaṇa as meaning either 'you gave her an excellent offspring', (su-prasavam) or 'you bestowed wealth on her' (aiśvarayam vā).]

You restored youth to the wise sage Kali, who was approaching old age (jaraṇām up eyushah); you raised Vandana from the well; and you made the maimed Vandana capable of moving about.(8)

Nirukta, 12, 1

The Aśvins are so called because they are everywhere (from root aśū, 'to spread'), one of them in the form of water (rasena) and the other in the form of light (jyotishā). The Aurṇanābhas, however, explain the word 'Aśvin' as meaning that they are possessors of horses (aśvaih). Who are these Aśvins? According to some, they symbolize earth and heaven (dyāvā pṛthivī); others see in them symbols of day and night (aho-rātrau); still others take them as sun and moon (sūryā-chandramasau). There are some (i.e., the aitihāsikas, historians) who regard them as meritorious princes (rājānau). One of them is the divinity of the heavenly firmament (dhyusthāna), and the other of the mid-region (madhya-sthāna).

Bṛhaddevatā, 6, 162,—

Tvashṭr had two children, a daughter, named Śaraṇyū and a son named Tri-Śiras. Śaranyū was given in marriage to Vivasvān. They begot twins, Yama and Yami. In due course, Śaraṇyū entrusted the care of the twins to another woman (whom she conjured up in her own image), and went away into wilderness (lit., disappeared). Vivasvān lived with this phantom woman and begot Manu. Later, he recognized the trick, and went in search of Śaraṇyū. She had in the meantime assumed the form of a mare and was wandering about. Vivasvān also assumed the form of a horse and won her affection. Their offsprings in this condition were the twins, Nāsatya and Dasra. They became celebrated as the Aśvins, 'the horse-divinities'.

II RUDRA AS PHYSICIAN

RV, 2, 33, —

O Rudra, we take care not to annoy you by our talk; and, O generous one (vṛshabha), we will not offend you by ignoble praises, nor by invoking other divinities. Invigorate us (or our children) by your medicinal herbs (bheshajebhih), for I hear you are the best among physicians (bhishaktamam).(4)

O Rudra, where is your famous hand that heals (bheshajah), that bestows happiness (jalāshah), and that delights (mṛlayākuh)? O generous one (vrshabha), you can rid even the gods of their distresses (rapasah)! Have mercy on me!(7)

RV, 5, 42,—

Praise him who has an unfailing arrow (svishuh), whose bow is mighty (sudhanvā), and who is the lord of all the healing herbs (viśvasya bheshajasya kshayati). Offer oblations to that Rudra for obtaining a strong and happy mind (mahe saumansāya). Prostrate before him who is an almighty god (asuram devam).(11)

III VARUṆA AS PHYSICIAN

RV, 1, 24, —

O governor, you have a hundred and a thousand medicines (bheshajah). May your compassionate mind (sumatih) be widespread (urvī) and majestic (gabhīra). Drive away the harmful spirit (Nirṛti, the demon of death) to a distant place, and rid us completely of the evil in us.(9)

O Mitra and Varuṇa, I take the Soma drink when the sun has just arisen; it heals the sick (āturasya bheshajam).(17)

IV SOMA AS HEALER

RV, 8, 79, —

Whatever is bare, he covers it. Whatever is sick (turam) he heals (bhishakti). (He makes) the blind see, and the lame walk.(2)

V AIR AS MEDICINE

RV, 10, 137, —

Wind (vāta), blow towards us the medicinal balm (bheshajam), and blow away from us the evil (repah, viz, disease). Truly are you the universal healer (viśvabheshaja), and messenger of the gods.(3)

VI WATER AS MEDICINE

RV, 10, 137, —

Water (āpa) indeed is a healer (bheshajī). Water destroys the diseases (amīvachātanīh), and water cures all (diseases) for all beings (sarvasya). May such water act as medicine to you, and make you happy.(6)

VII PHYSICIAN'S PROFESSION

RV, 9, 112, —

Various are our intentions, and various too are the vocations men follow. The carpenter seeks wood; the physician (bhishak) seeks diseases (rutam); the priest seeks to press the Soma juice. Flow on, Indu, for Indra!(1)

I am a singer; my father (or son) is a physician (bhishak), and my mother (or daughter) the grinder of corn. Different in our vocations, but (alike) desirous of wealth (vasuyavah), we have our place in the world. Flow on, Indu, for Indra!(2)

[**Note:** The word 'tatah' in the verse, according to Sāyaṇa means 'father', but Yāska explains that the word may mean either 'father' or 'son' for it has only the sense of procreation. Likewise 'nanā' may mean either 'mother' or 'daughter', according to Yāska (Nirukta, 6, 5), but 'mother' according to Sāyaṇa.

Both Yāska and Sāyaṇa give an alternate interpretation to the word 'bhishak', i.e., the master of ceremonies (brahmā) who corrects the errors or lapses and prescribes expiatory rites during the course of a sacrifice. But this is obviously a far-fetched interpretation, for the verse speaks of professions.]

VIII THE HYMN FOR MEDICINAL HERBS

RV, 10, 97, —

Long before (the appearance of) the

gods, even before the three ages (or seasons), were these ancient herbs (purvāh oshadhīh), bright-coloured and a hundred and seven in number. I recognize their abodes (i.e., uses).(1)

[**Note:** The expression tri-yugam is taken to mean either the three classical ages (Kṛta, Tretā and Dvāpara) or three seasons (summer, rains and winter) (Sāyaṇa). 'Bright-coloured' (babhrū) means 'invigorating' and 'exhilarating', like Soma. It also means 'nourishing' as food and as medicine. The antiquity of these medicinal plants is explained as being necessary nourishment for gods, humans and other animals. Food must be prior in existence to the animals that live on it.

The word oshadhi is explained by Yāska as 'destruction (dhayanti) of the defects or anomalies (oshat, i.e., dosha) in the body' (Nirukta, 9, 27). It also means what we ingest as food. Medicinal herbs are principally articles of food, which also cure diseases. These medicinal herbs are the divinities (devatā) that preside over this hymn (sūkta) consisting of twenty-three verses. The seer (ṛshi) of this hymn is 'the physician' (bhishak), son of Atharvana. Āśvalāyana-Śrauta-Sūtra (6, 9) explains that this hymn is to be employed if the participants in a sacrifice fall ill during the session.

The 'hundred and seven' abodes (śatam dhāmāni sapta cha) of these herbs may mean either innumerable places of origin (like mountains, plains, river-beds and forests) or innumerable shapes they are found in (like plants, shrubs, creepers, trees, bushes, flowering vegetation, fruit-yielding trees and so on); the 'abodes' may also mean 'names by which they are known and recognized' (Yāska).]

'Śatam sapta cha' may also mean 'seven hundred' and in this case, the reference is to the seven hundred vital points in the human body (marma-sthānas), on which the medicinal herbs act. Alternately, the expression may mean innumerable methods of preparation and application.

O dear mothers! A hundred (i.e., innumerable) are your places of origin (dhāmāni), and a thousand are the ways you grow (ruhah). O herbs that act in a hundred ways (śata-kratvah), make mine folk free from sickness (agadam kṛta).(2)

Rejoice ever, O herbs, bearing flowers and fruits in abundance, with branches spread alround, and, like horses, conquering disease (sajitvarih) and making all of us go beyond the clutches of distress (pārayishṇavah).(3)

I hail you, O herbs who are verily mothers! Physician, I give you horses and cows, clothes, and myself (i.e., my service).(4)

Your abode indeed is in the aśvattha tree and in the palāśa (parṇe) plant! When you take kindly to the physician (purusham savanatha), you render him wealthy (gobhāja, lit., givers of cattle to him).(5)

Where, O herbs, you have gathered together, like the princes in an assembly (samitau, 'on the battle-field' according to Sāyaṇa) the physician is called the wise sage (viprah), for he destroys the evil ones (rakshohā) and drives away diseases (amīvachātanah).(6)

I praise all the medicines (sarva-oshadhīh) the aśvavatī, the somavatī, the ūrjayantī, and the udojasa which dispel the diseases (asmai arishṭatātye).(7)

Like cows from the shed, O man, the energies of these medicinal herbs (oshadhīnām śushmāh) issue forth towards you, to render you wealthy (dhanam sanishyantīnām).(8)

Your mother is celebrated as 'the dispeller of all diseases' (ishkṛtih), and so are you all known, O herbs! You can indeed fly and move about! Heal, therefore, the sick (āmayati nishkṛtaḥ).(9)

Even as a thief enters the shed (and steals away the cows) all the herbs that are everywhere (parishthāh) attack the diseases, and take away whatever ailment is in the body (tanvah yat kiñcha rapah).(10)

When I hold in my hand these herbs (oshadhih haste ādadhe) for rendering the patient wholesome (vajayam) the strength of the disease (ātmā yakshmasya) withers away, even as the life of the birds when the hunter catches them.(11)

O herbs, like a valiant (monarch) in the midst of his army (madhyamaśir iva), you conquer the disease completely (yakshmam vibādhadhve) when you enter the (patient's body) from limb to limb, from joint to joint.(12)

Get lost at once, O disease, (flying fast) like the jay bird (chasha), (on the wings of) the blue jay (kikidivi), (departing) with the speed of wind, and (along) with the raging storm.(13)

O herbs, let each of you approach (avatu) the other, let each join with (upāvata) the other. Thus, all united (samvidānāh), fulfil my prayer (for health).(14)

May the herbs, brought well into being by Bṛhaspati (i.e., creator), (some) yielding fruits and (some) not, (some) producing flowers and (some) not, may these herbs free us from sickness (muñchantu amhasha).(15)

May the herbs free me from (the distress caused by) curses (śapathyāt); and from (the bonds of) Varuna. May they also free me from the fetters of Yama which hold back my feet (padbiśat), and from all the impurity with regard to the gods (devakilbishāt).(16)

Thus have the herbs, descending from the high heavens, declared: "He that is alive (jivam purushah) will not die (na rishyati), when we enter into him (aśnavāmahai).(17)

O herbs who have Soma for monarch, countless (bahvīh) and competent in a hundred ways (śata-vchashanāh) you are the best (uttama) among all the herbs! Be entirely bountiful (aram kāmāya), and a comfort to the heart (sam hṛde).(18)

O herbs, who have Soma for monarch, who have spread all over the earth (anu vishṭhitāh pṛthivim), and who have been brought forth by Bṛhaspati (i.e., creator), provide strength (sam datta vīryam), to this (sick person).(19)

May not he who digs the earth for you (khanitā) hurt you (mārishat); nor the person for whom I dig (yasmai khanāmi)! May the bipeds (i.e., human beings) and quadrupeds (cows, horses etc), and all beings be free from disease (anāturam astu).(20)

Let the plants that can listen to this prayer of mine as well as those that are far removed and not in sight (dūram parāgatāh), come together (sam-gatya) and bestow strength (sam-datta viryam) on this man (i.e., the patient).(21)

The herbs gather together and tell their monarch Soma: "O King, we will heal (pārayāmasi) him whom the knowledgeable physician (brāhmana) treats (kṛnoti)(22).

[**Note:** Sāyaṇa explains the word brāhmaṇa as 'the physician who is acquianted with the power of the herbs', i.e., drugs (oshadhīsāmarthyajñah vaidyah), and the word kṛṇoti as 'administers treatment (chikitsām karoti).

O herb, you are the best (among plants) (uttama); and all the plants (vṛkshāh, lit., trees) lie low before you (upastayah)! Let he who hurts us (i.e., the disease that attacks us), lie low before us!(23)]

[**Note:** This last verse is addressed to the Soma plant, according to Sāyaṇa. Soma is regarded as the divinity presiding over herbs and other plants. Soma is itself a plant, the exact identification of which is uncertain. There is an entire book of RV. (ninth maṇḍala) which is devoted to the glorification of Soma. The entire hymn is to be found also in Tattirīya-saṁhitā, 4,2,6. It appears that the hymn was employed not only during treatment of diseases by herbal medicine, but also during magic, sorcery and witchcraft.

IX ORIGIN OF ĀYURVEDA

CS, 1, 1, 3—34.

Bhāradvāja performed severe penances and desired long life. Guided by the sages he approached Indra, the monarch of the immortals. For Indra had obtained the 'science of life' (āyurveda) in its entirety from the Aśvins, who had got it from Daksha, who in turn had heard it from Brahma himself.

[**Note:** Brahma is the creator and the revealer of the Vedic lore. Daksha is his offspring, prajāpati, the 'lord of living beings' and the first of human governors. The Aśvins were the divine physicians who also came to the aid of human beings. Indra was a human hero, deified for his valour and achievements.]

When for human beings (those who were endowed with physical bodies) appeared diseases which obstructed their long life, austerities, study and exercise, the great and pious sages who were proficient in philosophical wisdom and experts in restraint over body and mind assembled on the slope of the Himālayan mountain, out of compassion for the living beings, and discussed (about diseases and their cure). Among those sages, filled with the lustre of penance and brilliant like the fire fed with clarified butter, were Angiras, Jamadagni, Vaśishtha, Kāśyapa, Bhrgu, Ātreya, Gautama, Sāṁkhya, Pulastya, Nārada, Asita, Agastya, Vāmadeva, Mārkaṇdeya, Āśvalāyana, Parīkshi, Bhikshu-Ātreya, Bharadvaja, Kapiñjala, Viśvāmitra, Āśmarathya, Bhārgava, Chyavana, Abhijit Gārgya, Śāṇḍilya, Kauṇḍinya, Varkshi, Devala, Gālava, Sānkṛtya, Baijavāpi, Kuśika, Bādarāyaṇa, Badiśa, Śaraloma, Kāpya, Kātyāyana, Śarkarāksha, Hiraṇyāksha, Lokāksha, Paingi, Śaunaka, Śakuneya, Maitreya, Maimatāyani, the Vaikhānasas and the Vālakhilyas.

They deliberated thus: "Health is the excellent source of the fulfilment of all human objectives: virtue, wealth and enjoyment. Diseases have now appeared striking at all these and threatening welfare and even life itself. This is indeed a great calamity for the human beings. What can possibly be the remedies for these ailments?" With this thought they contemplated for a while, and in their contemplative vision they beheld the help in Indra: "This monarch of the immortals would tell us the remedy!"

Then they considered who amongst them should be deputed to the abode of Indra to learn from him the remedy. The sage Bhāradvāja volunteered to undertake this task. Thereupon, having been deputed by them, Bhāradvāja went to where Indra resided and saw him glowing like fire, presiding over an assembly of the immortals. Having greeted him, Bhāradvāja communicated to him with humility the message that he had brought from the sages, viz., "Diseases have appeared, frightening all living beings. Tell me the remedy thereof".

Indra, ascertaining the enormous intellect of Bhāradvāja, expounded to him 'the science of life' (āyurveda) in short (or brief) words (padair alpaih) the causes (hetu), symptoms (linga) and therapeutics (aushadha) — this three-fold knowledge (trisūtram), which is enduring and meritorious, intent on the well-being of the healthy as well as the sick, as was learnt by the creator (Brahma). This science of life without limits, but in three branches (aetiology, symptomatology and therapeutics), was learnt by the sage Bhāradvāja promptly and quickly, for his mind was settled on it. Benefited greatly by this knowledge (lit., having secured long life and health), Bhāradvāja communicated this science to the other sages.

The sages obtained this science of enhancing the quality of life (vedam vardhanam āyushah) from Bhāradvāja in order to accomplish the well-being of all creatures (prajāhitam), and to prolong the life span (dīrgham āyuh). Putting into practice the prescriptions contained in this science, they obtained great happiness and long life.

[**Note:** The commentator Chkp discusses briefly the problem of Ātreya-Punarvasu. He cities a view, which he rejects as incorrect, that Ātreya was another name of Bhāradvāja. He also cites *Hārīta-saṁhitā* to the effect that Ātreya was a disciple of Bhāradvāja: the lineage here assumes this form: Indra-Bhāradvāja-Ātreya-Hārīta. Vāgbhaṭa's remark that Indra taught this science to Atriputra (viz., Ātreya) (Ahr, 1,1,3) merely suggests that Indra had several students besides Bhāradvāja.]

Agniveśa had exceptional brilliance and so he was the first to compose a treatise (tantra) on what he learnt, and not because he had received any special instructions from the teacher (Punarvasu-Ātreya). Then the wise ones like Bhela and others prepared their own treatises and presented them to the teacher (Punarvasu-Ātreya). These treatises were very well received by the assembly of sages, who not only approved but praised the works as contributing to the welfare of all creatures.

[**Note:** Agniveśa's treatise (tantra) forms the source book for *Charaka-saṁhitā.*]

SS, 1, 1, 2—4

When (long-ago) Divodāsa-Kāśi-rāja, who was none other than the reverend Dhanvantari the best among the immortals, was seated surrounded by hosts of gods and sages, in his own hermitage, Aupadhenava, Vaitarana, Aurabhra, Paushkalāvata, Karvīrya, Gopurarakshita, Suśruta and others approached him, and said: "Revered master, we are troubled in mind when we behold human beings, who even though well equipped and attended in life, yet are oppressed by diseases, physical, mental, and accidental, and suffer helplessly much agony. We would therefore desire to be instructed by you in the 'science of life' (āyurveda) by means of which we may relieve their sufferings in order to help them seek for happiness in life; we may also, incidentally, attend to our own health in life (prāṇayātrārtham). Because welfare in this world as well as in the world beyond is dependent upon this science (atrāyattam aihikam āmushmikam cha śreyah), we have come to you to be instructed by you in that science."

To them, the revered master replied: "Welcome to all of you. You are indeed worthy of being instructed in this discipline!"

BP, 'Pūrva-khaṇḍa', 1, 2-17

I shall first of all write about how this 'science of life' (āyurveda) appeared on earth; and I have consulted many treatises on this matter. Āyurveda is the science in which life, what helps it and what hurts it, how disease is caused and how it is cured, are dealt with. The human being knows about good life and obtains it through this science; and it is therefore that sages call it Āyurveda.

The creator, purporting to reveal the essential import of Atharva-veda, composed in his own name a lucid treatise (saṁhitā) consisting of one lakh verses. Then he, the veritable ocean of wisdom, instructed this science with all its branches to Daksha, who was an adept in all activities. Later Daksha taught it to the twin-gods (the aśvins), children of Sūrya and noblest among the gods, who became physicians of the gods (suravaidyāh). Having received instructions from Daksha, these Aśvins prepared their own treatise (samhitām svīyām), to enhance the knowledge of all physicians. (The exploits of the Aśvins are narrated in verses 9-14.) By these activities the best among the physicians, the Aśvins, became objects of adoration for Indra and other gods.

Indra, beholding the beneficial treatment effected by them, earnestly begged them to impart to him this science. Thereupon, the

Aśvins taught Indra the science as they had learnt it. Then Indra communicated what he had got from the Aśvins to several sages headed by Ātreya.

[Note: What follows is an account of how Indra came to impart the wisdom of Āyurveda to Ātreya (verses 18-34).]

Once, the revered sage Ātreya happened to perceive here and there that people were afflicted with diseases, and he began to deliberate: "What shall I do? Where shall I go? How can these folk be free from diseases? I cannot rest in peace when I look at their suffering. I am by nature kind-hearted, and nature cannot be foresaken! When these people suffer, I too begin to suffer! I shall study Āyurveda for relieving the folk of their ailments."

Having thus resolved, Ātreya went to the dwelling of the immortals. He beheld there Indra, seated on his throne and being eulogized by the sages: he was brilliant like the sun, illumining the ten quarters; he was the great teacher of Āyurveda, and therefore was adored by the immortals. When Indra saw Ātreya entering, he at once came down from his throne and greeted the sage in all humility. He made kind inquiries, and implored to be told the reason of the sage's visit. Ātreya replied: "O monarch of the gods, you are the ruler not only of the heavenly realms, but of all the three worlds, for so the creator ordained. The world of human beings is afflicted by diseases, and the people are sorely distressed. There is grief on earth, and you must take pity on the living beings. Have compassion on the people and teach me the 'science of life' (āyurveda)

Indra agreed and instructed the sage in the 'science of life' in all its branches (sāngam); and the sage returned to earth, having blessed the monarch of the gods.

Then Ātreya, supreme among sages and most compassionate, composed a treatise in his own name (sva-nāmnā samhitām chakre), for the welfare of the entire mankind. He taught this treatise to Agniveśa, Bhela, Jatūkarṇa, Parāśara, Kshīrapāṇi and Hārīta.

Agniveśa was the first to prepare a manual (tantra) based on this instruction, followed by Bhela and others with their own manuals. They all read their manuals in the presence of Ātreya amidst the assembly of sages. Ātreya was happy at these writings and congratulated them. The sages and the gods too were delighted.

[Note: Then follows an account concerning Bhāradvāja in verses 35-56.]

Once, on the slope of the Himālayan mountain, a large number of sages had gathered: Bhāradvāja was the first among them, then Angiras, Garga, Marīchi, Bhṛgu, Bhārgava, Pulastya, Agasti, Asita, Vaśishṭha, Parāśara, Hārīta, Gautama, Sāṁkhya, Maitreya, Chyavana, Jamadagni, Kāśyapa, Gargya, Kaśyapa, Nārada, Vāmadeva, Mārkaṇḍeya, Kapiñjala, Śāṇḍilya, Kauṇḍinya, Śakuneya, Śaunaka and others.

They deliberated amongst themselves: The body alone is truly the source of virtue, wealth, enjoyment and liberation. If it becomes free from diseases, all the above objectives would be fulfilled; but if it is oppressed by disease then penance, study, virtuous conduct, vows of celibacy and even life would be obstructed. Diseases emaciate the body, diminish the vigour, render activity difficult, rob the sense-organs of their function and cause pain to the entire body. They not only forcibly impede our striving, for virtue, wealth, enjoyment and liberation, but quickly take away life itself. How can beings be happy (when diseases abound)? Therefore, the wise among you must think of some means by which diseases are eliminated. Then they addressed Bhāradvāja: "You amongst us are the most suitable. You approach Indra and obtain from him the 'science of life' (āyurveda), which has come to him in a lineage (labdham kramāt). By studying it, we will become free from the fear of diseases!"

[**Note:** Then follows the account of his visit to Indra as found in *CS,* 1,1,20-29. In verse 57 begins the story of Charaka which continues till verse 65.]

When (in the distant past) the Vedic lore was extricated by Vishṇu (Hari) in his incarnation as Fish, Śesha (Vishṇu's serpentine attendant) obtained a knowledge of the Veda in all its branches and with all the aids of study (vedam sāngam). And (at that very time) he secured 'the science of life' (āyurveda) which was included in the Atharva-corpus (atharvāntargatam).

Once he came down in the guise of a wanderer (chara) to acquaint himself with the affairs of the world of human beings. He saw people afflicted by diseases and torn with sorrow; he found people here and there agitated, and about to die. He was overcome by compassion for them; and their misery filled him with grief. He then deliberated upon the means of relieving the folk of their maladies.

He became the son of a sage, Viśuddha by name, who was celebrated as learned in the Vedic lore. He came here like a wanderer, and no one knew whence he had come. Therefore he became known in the world as 'the wanderer' (Charaka). He, this 'preceptor Charaka', shines in the world as the preceptor of the gods shines in heaven; an incarnation of Sesha (Ananta), who healed the diseases of mankind. He collected and redacted the treatises (tantrāṇi samskṛtya samāhṛtya) of Agniveśa and others who were disciples of the sage Atreya, and prepared a manual in his own name.

[**Note:** Then follows the account of Dhanvantari in verses 66-75.]

Once Indra, the monarch of gods, turned his attention to the world below, and found mankind grievously afflicted with diseases. His heart was overcome, by compassion, and, taking pity on mankind, he addressed Dhanvantari thus: "O revered Dhanvantari, supreme among the immortals, listen to me! You are competent, and therefore help the living beings. What has not been done in times of yore to benefit the world? Vishṇu, the lord of the three realms, assumed several incarnations such as the Fish. Therefore, go to the world and become a King in the Kāśi region. And reveal 'the science of life' (āyurveda), in order to combat the diseases!"

So saying, the master of the gods, imparted the entire 'science of life' (āyushovedam) to Dhanvantari, with a desire to contribute to the welfare of all living beings. Having mastered the medical lore under Indra, Dhanvantari came down to the earth and was born in the household of Bāhuja (kshatriya). He became known to people as Divodāsa.

Even as a boy, he renounced the pleasures of life and wandered about, performing great austerities. With great difficulty, Brahma (the creator) persuaded him to become the King of Kāśi. From then on, Dhanvantari became celebrated among people as 'Kāśi-rāja' ('the monarch of Kāśi') For securing the welfare of living beings, he composed his own treatise (saṁhitā), and taught it to students.

[**Note:** Then follows an account of Suśruta in verses 76-85.]

Then by their powers of supernatural intuition, the sages headed by Viśvāmitra learnt that Dhanvantari had appeared on earth as Kāśi-rāja in the Kāśi region. Viśvāmitra beckoned his son and told him: "Dear one, go to the city of Kāśi, graced by the presence of the Lord of All (Viśveśvara). There is a kshatriya there by the names of Divodāsa and Kāśi-rāja. He is in reality Dhanvantari himself, the foremost among the masters of the 'science of life'. Learn from him this 'science of life' for the sake of helping mankind (lokopakṛtihetave). The most sacred spot to visit (tīrtha) is compassion for all living beings (sarva-prāṇidayā); and the most meritorious sacrifice is benefaction (upakāra)."

Heeding to the words of his father, Suśruta came to Kāśi, along with a hundred youths who were all children of sages. They approached in humility the venerable Dhanvantari, who had then been dwelling as an anchorite in a hermitage (vānaprasthāśrame), surrounded by many sages. When the supreme among the gods, Dhanvantari-Divodāsa welcomed them, and inquired why they had come, Suśruta as their spokesman said: "Revered Sir, beholding human beings tormented by diseases, and being in the grip of sorrow and despair, our own hearts are overcome with sorrow. We have come here to learn from you the means of relieving their distress. Kindly instruct us in the 'science of life'."

The royal sage agreed and taught them. When the delighted sages finished their period of learning, they blessed the royal sage and returned to their homes. Suśruta, among them, was the first to prepare his own manual on these teachings (svatantram); his friends also (later) composed their own manuals. The manual of Suśruta was studied widely, and therefore it was truly 'well-read' (Suśruta) and that is how it has become celebrated in the world.

Select Bibliography

Select Bibliography

Antū-bhāi-vaidya, *Vanaspati-parichay,* Bombay, Ayurveda Research Inst., 1952.

Āyurveda-mahodadhi (Sushena-vaidyaka), (S) Bombay, Venkateshvara Press, 1915.

Banerjee, D.N., *Āyurveda-Śārīa* (S), Calcutta, 1951

Basava, *Basava-rājīyaṁ,* (S), Madras, V. Ramaswami Sastrulu and Sons, 1951.

Bhagvat-Sinhjee, *A Short History of Äryan Medical Sciences,* London, 1896.

Bhagavan Dash, *Ayurvedic Treatment for Common Diseases,* New Delhi 1975.

Bhagavan Dash and Lalitesh Kashyap, *Materia Medica of Āyurveda,* New Delhi, Concept Publ., Co. 1980

Bhagvan Dash, *Tibetan Medicine,* Dharamsala, Lib. Tib. Works and Arch., 1976.

Bhaishajya-ratnāvalī, (S), N.N. Mitra (ed), Delhi, Motilal Banarsidass, 1962.

Bhāva-miśra, *Bhāva-prakāśa,* (S), Jivananda Vidyasagar (ed), 1875.

Bhela, *Bhela Saṁhitā, (S), Asutosh Mookerjee (ed), Calcutta, Calcutta Univ., 1921.*

Bhoja, Rasa-rāja-mṛgāṅka (S), Bombay, Y.T. Acharya (ed), 1923.

Binodlal Sen, *Āyurveda-vijñana,* (S), 2 vols, Calcutta, 1887

Bose, D.M. et al (ed), *A Concise History of Science in India,* New Delhi, Indian National Science Academy, 1971.

Bower Manuscripts (S), A.F.R. Hoernle (ed), Calcutta, 1909 (Parts I-VII, Calcutta 1893-7).

Chakrapāṇi-datta, *Chikitsā-sāra-saṁgraha,* (S) Calcutta, Jivananda Vidyasagara, 1888.

Chakrapāni-datta, *Dravya-guṇa-saṁgraha,* (S), Calcutta, 1871.

Chāmuṇḍa, *Rasa-Saṅketa-Kalikā.*(S), Bombay, Y.T. Acharya, 1912.

Charaka, *Rasa-saṅketa- Kalikā,* (S), Bombay, Y.T. Acharya, 1912.

Charaka, *Charaka-saṁhitā,* (S) (with comm. of Chakrapāṇi-datta), Bombay, Nirnaya Sagar 1941; Jamnagar, Gulab Kunverba Ayurvedic Society, 1949 (6 vol).

Chattopadhyaya, Debiprasad, *Science and Society in Ancient India,* Calcutta, Research India Publ., 1977.

Chopra, R.N., *Glossary of Indian Medicinal Plants,* New Delhi, CSIR, 1956.

Chūdāmaṇi, *Rasa-Kāmadhenu,* (S) Bombay, Y.T. Acharya (ed), 1925; Gondal, Jivaram Kalidas, 1925.

Dalhaṇa, *Nibanda-saṁgraha,* (S), Calcutta, Jivananda Vidyasagar (ed), 1891.

Dasgupta, S.N., *A History of Indian Philosophy,* vol II, ch. XIII, "Speculations in the Medical Schools", Cambridge, The Syndics of Cambridge Univ. Press, 1932.

Devadatta, *Dhātu-ratna-mālā,* (S), Poona, 1914.

Dhārākalpa, Y.T. Acharya (ed), Bombay 1923.

Dutta, U.C., *The Materia Medica of the Hindus,* Calcutta 1870, Varanasi, Chowkhamba, 1980 (Revised third ed).

Filliozat, J., *The Classical Doctrine of Indian Medicine,* Delhi, Munshi Ram Manohar Lal, 1964.

Finckh, Elisabeth, *Foundations of Tibetan Medicine,* London and Watkins, Watkins, 1978.

Gopāla-Kṛshṇa, *Rasendra-saṁgraha,* (S), Varanasi, Chowkhamba Skt. Series, 1937.

Govinda, *Rasa-hṛdaya,* (S), Bombay, Y.T. Acharya (ed), 1911.

Gupta, Umesh-Chandra, *Vaidyaka-śabda-sindhu,* (S), Calcutta, 1894.

Iyer, T.G. Ramamurti, *The Handbook of Indian Medicine or The Gems of Siddha System,* Erode, Sri Vani Vilas Press, 1933.

Jolly, J., *Early Medical Literature of India,* London 1893.

Jolly, J., *Indian Medicine,* Tr. by C.G. Kashikar, Poona, 1951; Delhi Munshi Ram Manohar Lal, 1977.

Jivanrām Vaidya; *Forceps used by the Ancients of India,* Bombay 1892.

Kālidas, Jīvarām, *Rasa-chintāmaṇi* (S), Bombay, 1914.

Kāśīnātha, *Ajīrṇa-mañjarī,* (S) mss.

Kāśyapa-saṁhitā, (S), (on Toxicology) Yatirāja-Svāmī (ed), Madras, 1933.

Kāśyapa-saṁhitā, (S) (On Midwifery and Gynaecology), Y.T. Acharya and Hemaraj Sarma, Bombay, Nirnaya-Sagar, 1938.

Keśava, *Siddha-mantra-prakāśa,* (S), Bombay, Y.T. Acharya, 1909.

Kutumbiah, P, *Ancient Indian Medicine,* Madras, Orient Longmans, 1962.

Lal-Sengupta, K.B., *Āyurveda-dravyābhidhāna,* (S), Calcutta, 1895.

Lolambarāja, *Vaidyāvataṁsa,* Ahmedabad, 1908.

Lolambarāja, *Vaidya-jīvana,* Bombay, Venkateshvar Press, 1910.

Mādhava, *Āyurveda-prakāśa* (S), Yadavji Trikumji (ed), Bombay, 1924.

Mādhava, *Prayoga-chintāmaṇi,* (S), Calcutta.

Mādhava-kara, *Rugviniśchaya, (Mādhava-nidāna)* (S) (with comm. of Vijaya-rakshita and Srikantha), Sarada Charana Sen (ed), Varanasi, 1932; Y.T. Acharya (ed), Bombay 1920; with Madhu Kosha, Jivananda, Calcutta 1875.

Mitra-miśra, *Vīramitrodaya* (S), Calcutta, Jivananda Vidyasagara (ed), 1875.

Mookerjee, Bhudev, *Rasa-jala-nidhi,* (S), Calcutta, 1926.

Moreśvara, *Vaidyāmṛta,* (S), Varanasi, 1867.

Mukhopadhyay, B., *History of Indian Medicine,* (3 vols), Calcutta, Calcutta Univ., 1922-29).

Mukhopadhyay, G., *Surgical Instruments of the Hindus,* Calcutta.

Nadkarni, K.M., *Indian Materia Medica* (2 vols), Bombay, Popular Prakashan, 1976 (3rd ed).

Nakula, *Aśva-chikitsā* (S), Calcutta, Bibl. Ind., 1886.

Nārāyaṇa, *Rāja-vallabha-dravya-guṇa* (S), Bombay, Venkateshwar Press.,

Nighaṇṭu-ratnākara (S) Godbole (ed), Bombay 1867.

Pārada-kalpa (Rudra-yāmala) (S), (2 vols), Bombay, Y.T. Acharya (ed), 1911 and 1915.

Pārishadyam Śabdārtha-śarīram (S), Damodar Sharma Gaud (ed), Nagpur, Vaidyanath Ayurved Bhavan, 1979.

Rāma, Vaidyaka-sāra (S), Bombay, Raghuvamsa Sarma, 1896.

Rāvaṇa, *Arka-prakāśa,* (S), Bombay, Venkatesvara Press, Madras, D. Gopalacharlu (ed), 1914.

Rāvaṇa, *Nāḍī-parīkshā,* (S), Bombay, Y. T. Acharya (ed) 1923.

Ray, P. and Gupta, H. N. *Charaka-saṁhitā:* A Scientific Synopsis, New Delhi, Ind. National Science Academy, 1965.

Ray, P., Gupta H. N., and Roy, M: *Suśruta-saṁhitā, A Scientific Synoposis,* New Delhi, Ind. National Science Academy, 1980.

Ray, P. C. *History of Hindu Chemistry,* (2 vols), Calcutta 1902 and 1925.

Rechung Rimpoche, *Tibetan Medicine,* Berkeley, Univ. of California Press, 1973.

Royle, An *Essay on the Antiquity of Hindu Medicine,* London, 1837.

Śālinātha, *Rasa-mañjarī* (S), Poona, T. G. Kale, 1915.

Śaṅkara, *Vaidya-vinoda,* (S), Bombay, Venkateshvar Press, 1913.

Śārṅgadhara-saṁhitā, (S), Prabhu-ram Jivan-ram (ed), Bombay, 1891; Bombay, Nirnaya-Sagara, 1922.

Savanur, H. V.; *A Handbook of Ayurvedic Materia Medica,* vol I, Belgaum, Jathar, 1950.

Seal, B. N. *Positive Sciences of the Ancient Hindus,* Calcutta.

Sen, Gaṇanāth, *Pratyaksha-śārīram,* (S), Part I, Calcutta 1913.

Sengupta, N. N.: *The Ayrvedic System of Medicine,* vol I, Calcutta, 1919.

Sharma, P, V.; *Āyurved ka* vaijñānik itihās, Banaras, 1975.

Sharma, P. V., Dravya-guṇa-*vaijñanaṁ,* (S), Varanasi, Chowkhamba Skt. Sansthān 1978 (- vols).

Siegerist, H. E.: *A History of Medicine* (2 vols), Yale, 1951-61.

Soḍhala, *Gada-nigraha,* (S), Y. T. Acharya, Bombay 1924.

Śrībindu, *Rasa-paddhati,* (S), Y. T. Acharya, Bombay, 1925.

Suśruta, *Suśruta-saṁhitā,* (S), Calcutta Jīvānanda Vidyasagara (ed), 1889; (with *Bhānumati* and *Nibandha-saṁgraha),* Calcutta, Ganga-prasad Sen (ed), 1888 ff; Bombay, Nirnaya-Sagara, 1915 and 1931; Calcutta, N.N. Sengupta and B.C. Sengupta 1937 (2 vols).

Tīsaṭa, *Chikitsā-Kalikā,* (S), (with comm. of Chandraṭa), Lahore, Mitra Ayurvedic Pharmacy, 1926; Kottayam, N. S. Moos, 1950

Toḍarānanda, (S), Bikaner, Anup Skt. Lib.

Trimalla, *Yoga-taraṅgiṇī,* (S), Poona, Ānandāśrama Sanksrit Series, 1913.

Udupa, K. N., and Singh R.H., *Science and Philosophy of Indian Medicine,* Nagpur, Baidyanath, 1978.

Ugrāditya, *Kalyāṇa-kāraka,* (S), Sholapur, 1940.

Vāgbhaṭa: *Ashṭāṅga-hṛdaya* (S), Bombay, G.K. Press, 1880; Jivananda Vidyasagara (ed), Calcutt, 1882; A. M. Kunte (ed), Bombay 1891; Motilal Banarsidass, Lahore, 1933; (with comm. of Chandranandana, Aruṇa-datta and Hemādri), Bombay, Venkateshvara Press, 1928; (with comm. of Aruṇadatta and Hemādri), Bombay, Nirnaya-Sagar, 1939; (with comm. of Parameśvara), Kottayam, N. S.

Moos, 1950; (with Hindu tr. after Sarvāṅga-sundara), Banaras, Motilal Banarsidass 1963.

Vābhaṭa, *Rasa-ratna-samucchaya,* (S), Poona, Ānandāśrama Skt. Series, 1890; Calcutta (with Bengali tr.), 1915.

Vallabha, *Vaidya-chintāmaṇi,* (S), Madras, P. V. K. Rao, 1921.

Vaṅgasena, *Chikitsā-sāra-saṁgraha,* (S), Calcutta, Jivananda Vidyasagara, 1893; Lahore, 1928.

Vararuchi, *Yoga-śataka,* (S) with Sinhalese Comm., Colombo, M.P. Parera, 1877.

Vîra-rājendra, *Sakala-vaidya-samhitā-sārārṇava,* Mysore,Mysore Univ., 1932 and 1964.

Vṛnda, *Siddha-yoga,* (S), (with comm. of Śrî-kaṇṭha), Poona, 1894

Vṛnda-madhava, (S), Poona, Hanumant-Sastri Padhye, 1894.

Webb, A., *The Historical Relations of Ancient Hindu with Greek Medicine,* Calcutta, 1850.

Wilson H.H.: *On the Medical and Surgical Sciences of the Hindus,* Calcutta, 1845; London 1864.

Wise, T.A., *Commentary on the Hindu System of Medicine,* Calcutta, 1845; London 1860.

Yādavji-Trikamji Āchārya, *Ḍravya-guṇa-vijñānaṁ,* (S) (2 vols), Nagpur, Vaidyanath Ayurved Bhavan, 1976.

Yaśodhara, *Rasa-prakāśa-sudhākara,* (S), Gondal, Jivaram Kalidas, 1926.

Yogānanda-nātha, *Āyurveda-sūtra,* (S), Mysore, University of Mysore, 1922.

Zimmer, H.R., *Hindu Medicine,* Balimore, John Hopkins, 1948.

Specimen Pages of Language Texts

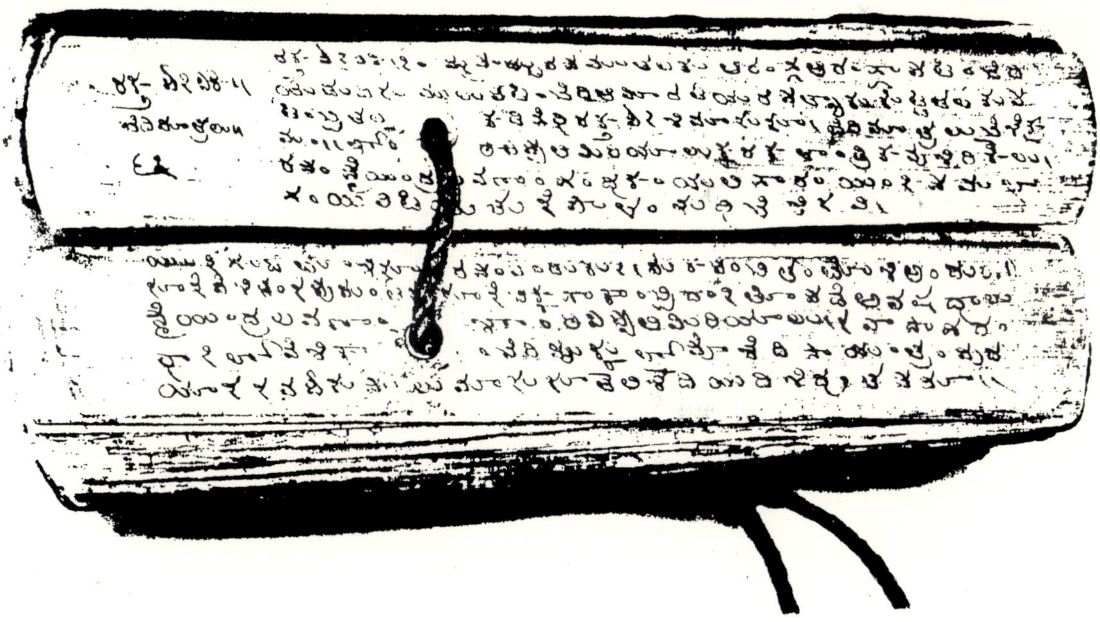

Specimen of a Palm-leaf manuscript of recipes prepared by the physicians.

టీ॥ కిరాతతిక్తః-కైరాతః-భూనింబః-రామసేనకః-అనునవి నేలవేము పేర్లు.
[நிலவேம்பு=నిలవేంబు]

నేలవేముగుణము.

శ్లో॥ భూనింబో వాతలస్స్నిగ్ధః కఫపిత్తజ్వరాపహః । వ్రణసంతాపణః పథ్యః కుష్ఠకండూతిశోఫహృత్ ॥

తా॥ నేలవేము వాతముజేసును జిగటగనుండును కఫజ్వరము పిత్తజ్వరము వ్రణములు కుష్టువు దురద వాపు వీటినిపోగొట్టును. పథ్యకరముగ నుండును.

తురకవేము.

శ్లో॥ కిరాతకోన్యో నైపాలో నాడితిక్తో జ్వరాంతకః । కండుతిక్తోర్ధతిక్తస్స్యాత్సన్నిద్రారిస్సన్నిపాతహా॥

టీ॥ నైపాలః-నాడితిక్తః-జ్వరాంతకః-కండుతిక్తః-అర్ధతిక్తః-నిద్రారిః సన్నిపాతహా-అనునవి తురకవేము పేర్లు. [மலைவேம்பு=మలైవేంబు]

తురకవేముగుణము.

శ్లో॥ నైపాలో వాతలోరూక్షశ్శీతలస్తిక్తకో లఘుః। సన్నిపాతజ్వరశ్వాసకాసపిత్తాస్రదాహనుత్ । కఫపిత్తంజ్వరంకుష్ఠంకండూంశోఫంకృమీన్ జయేత్ ॥

తా॥ తురకవేము వాతముజేసును. తాపమునిచ్చును. శీతలముగ చేదుగనుండును. తేలికనిచ్చును. సన్నిపాతజ్వరము శ్వాసము కాసము పిత్తరక్తము అంగతాపము కఫము పిత్తము జ్వరము కుష్టువు దురద వాపు నులిపురుగులు వీటిని హరింపజేయును.

కరివేప.

శ్లో॥ కైడర్యోథమహానింబో రావణో గిరినిమ్బకః॥

టీ॥ కైడర్యః-మహానింబః-రావణః-గిరినింబకః-అనునవి కరివేపపేర్లు.
[கறிவேப்பை=కరివేప్పై]

కరివేపగుణము.

శ్లో॥ కైడర్యః కటుకస్తిక్తః కషాయశ్శీతలో లఘుః । సంతాపశోఫకుష్ఠార్శః క్రిమిభూతవిషాపహా॥

తా॥ కరివేప కారముగ చేదుగ వగరుగ శీతలముగనుండును. తేలికనిచ్చును. దేహతాపము శోష కుష్టువు మూలము క్రిములు భూతములవలనిబాధ విషము వీటినిపోగొట్టును.

Oshadhi-guṇa-mañjari, a glossary of medicinal herbs in Sanskrit and Telugu, prepared by Īchambādi Śrīnivāsāchārya, and printed in Madras in 1912, included in *Sarvaushadhi-guṇa-kalpamu*.

॥ श्री ॥

शार्ङ्गधरसंहिता.

श्रीगणेशायनमः॥ ॥ग्रंथाचे आरंभीं मध्यें आणि शेवटीं मंगल असावें असें शास्त्र व शिष्टाचार आहे यास्तव ग्रंथाकार शिवभवानीस्मरणरूप मंगल करितात.

श्रियंसदद्यादृवतांपुरारिर्यदंगतेजःप्रसरेभवा- मंगलाचरण.
नी॥विराजतेनिर्मलचंद्रिकायांमहौषधीवज्व-
लिताहिमाद्रौ॥१॥ ॥छ॥ ॥छ॥

अर्थ.– हिमालयाच्या ठायीं अत्यंत देदीप्यमान महौषधी चंद्रज्योत्स्ना असतां जशी शोभा पावत्ये त्या प्रकारें ज्याचे अंगतेजःप्रसाराचे ठायीं भवानी शोभते असा जो शिव तो तुह्मास लक्ष्मीतें देवो.

प्रसिद्धयोगामुनिभिःप्रयुक्ताश्चिकित्सकैर्येबहुशो- ग्रंथालासम्म
नुभूताः॥विधीयतेशार्ङ्गधरेणतेषांसःसंग्रहःसज्ज- त्त व ग्रंथा
नरंजनाय॥२॥ चें प्रयोजन.

अर्थ.– चरकादिक मुनीनी कथन केलें आणि वैद्यानीं वारंवार नाम रूप योजनादिके करून अनुभविले असे जे विख्यात योग त्यांचा सुसंग्रह साधूंचे मनोरंजनार्थ शार्ङ्गधराचार्य कथन करितात.

हेत्वादिरूपाकृतिसात्म्यजातिभेदैःसमीक्ष्यातु- रोगनिश्चय
रसर्वरोगान्॥ चिकित्सितंकर्षणबृंहणाख्यंकु- पूर्वकचिकि
र्वीतवैद्योविधिवत्सुयोगैः॥३॥ ॥छ॥ त्सा.

अर्थ.– हेतु आदिरूपें आकृति सात्म्यें जाती या भेदें करून रोग्यांचे-

The first page of *Śārṅgadhara-Saṃhitā*, an early lithographic edition issued from Bombay in 1877.

१४६

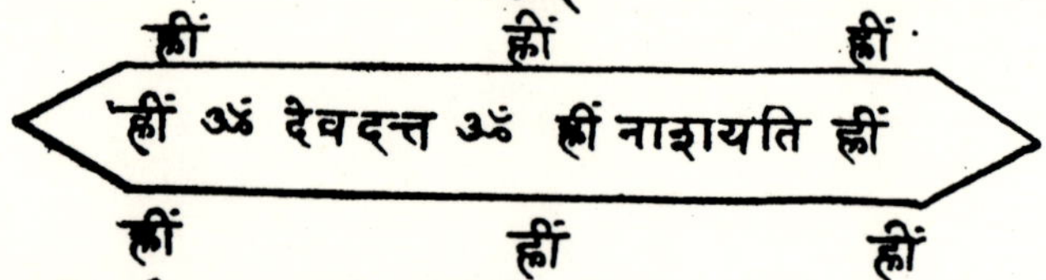

गोरोचनसे भोजपत्रपर लिख पात्रमें रख दूधसे प्लावित कर जलमें डालदे शत्रुकी शांति हो.

१४७

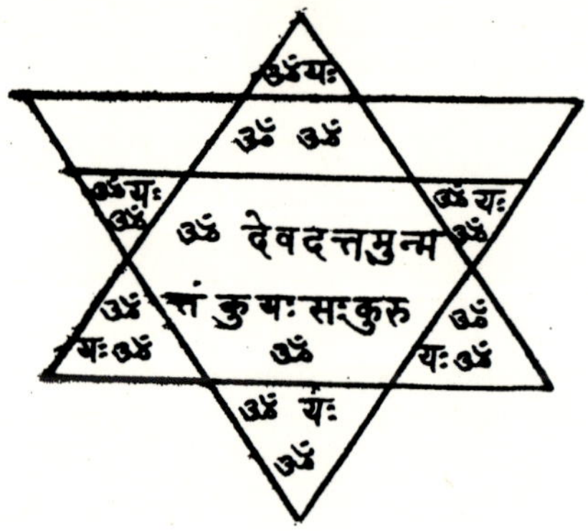

धतूरेके रस और काकके रुधिरसे उद्भ्रान्त पत्रपर लिख नीमकी शाखामें वायव्य दिशामें धारणकरे तो उन्मत्त हो यह अनुभव किया है सत्य है.

१४८

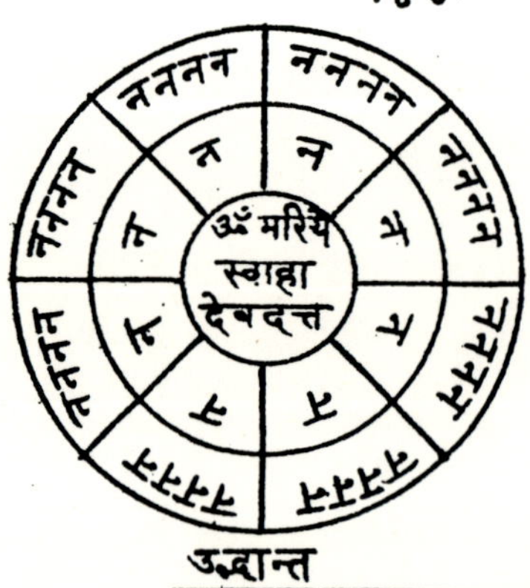

उद्भ्रान्त

भोजपत्रसे इष्टवा हरिद्रा हरितालसे जिसका नाम लिख प्रच्छन्न स्थापन करे वह नष्ट हो निकालनेसे स्वस्थ हो.

Pages from a Tantrik text, giving alchemic, herbal, and magical cures, *Kāma-ratnam* hand-printed by litho process in Bombay (Lakshmi-Venkateshwar Press) in 1824.

मंत्रश्रौर यंत्र दोनोंहीकें करनेसे शीघ्र सिद्धि होती है· निजनिज विधिके मंत्र विधिसे समझलेना

१५०

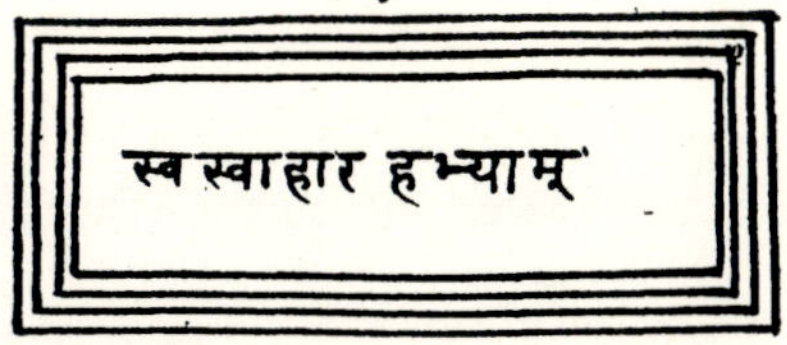

साध्यके रक्तसे शत्रु कानाम भोजपत्रपर लिख सिकोरेमें डाल ज्वलित अग्निमें स्थापन करे उसी समय शत्रु नष्ट हो·

१४९

पाताल यंत्र

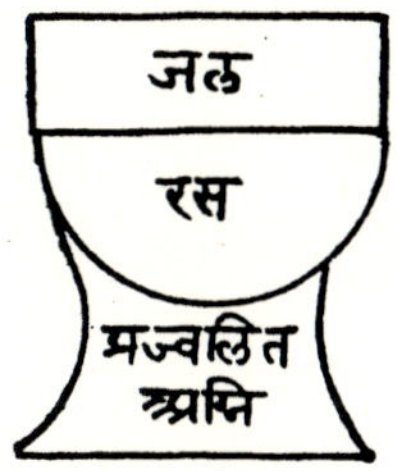

१५१

वालुका यंत्र·

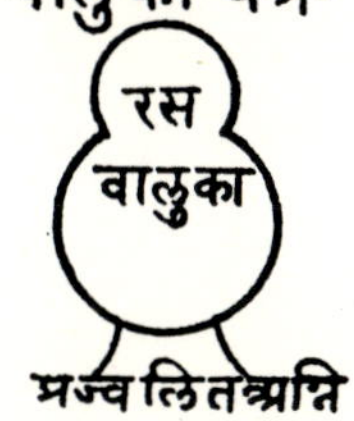

दोला यंत्र

१५२

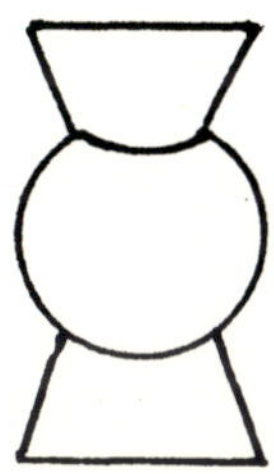

कच्छप यंत्र १५३

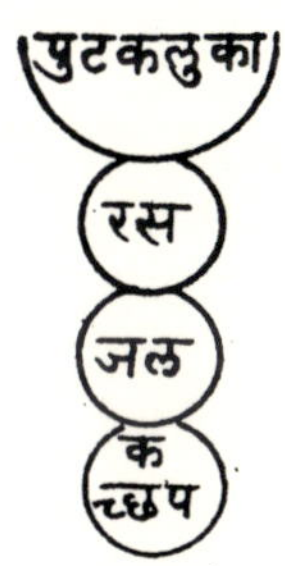

१५५

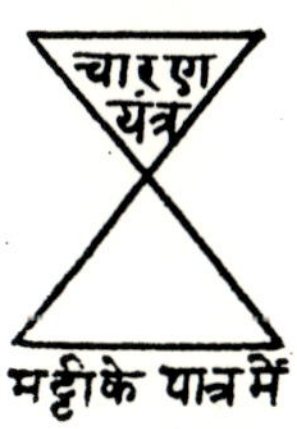

१५४

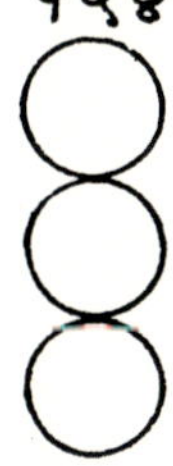

भूधर यंत्र·

इति कामरत्न परिशिष्टम्.

शलाकाशस्त्रम्।

ताम्री शलाका द्विमुखा मुखे कुररकाकृतिः।
नेत्रनाड़ीं तथा विध्येत् कफदोषसमुद्भवाम्॥

मुद्रिका।

प्रदेशिन्यग्रपर्व्वप्रमाणा फलेऽर्द्धाङ्गुलायता मुद्रिका।

वड़िशः।

अक्ष्णो शुण्डिकार्मादेर्वड़िशः सुनताननः।

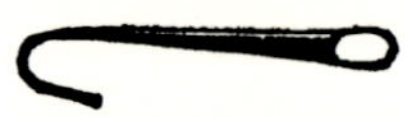

करपत्रम्।

भेदेऽस्थ्नां करपत्रन्तु खरधारं दशाङ्गुलम्।
विस्तारे द्व्यङ्गुलं सूक्ष्मदन्तं सत्सरुबन्धनम्॥

कर्त्तरी।

स्नायुस्थिगर्भशल्यानां केशादीनाञ्च कर्त्तने।
विविधाकृतयो योज्याः कर्त्तर्य्यः कर्त्तरीनिभाः॥

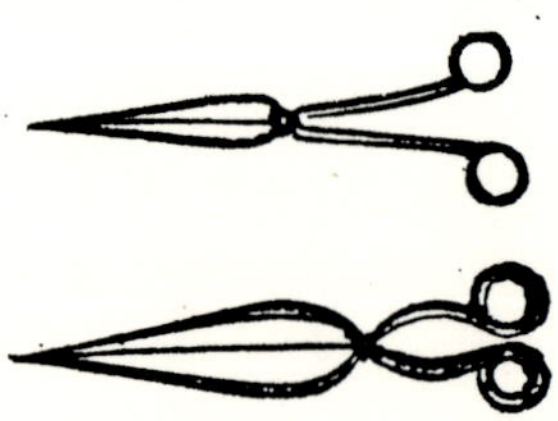

Specimen pages of illustrations of surgical instruments described by Suśruta, given by an early Āyurvedic treatise in Sanskrit, *Āyurveda-vijnānam* by Vinod Lal Sengupta, Calcutta, printed in the year 1927.

अधिकन्तु विषघ्नोऽयम्। अस्य त्वग्ग्राह्या, मात्रा १ माषकः। लोध। पटियालोध। सावरलोध।

प्रियङ्गुर्गन्धप्रियङ्गुश्च ।

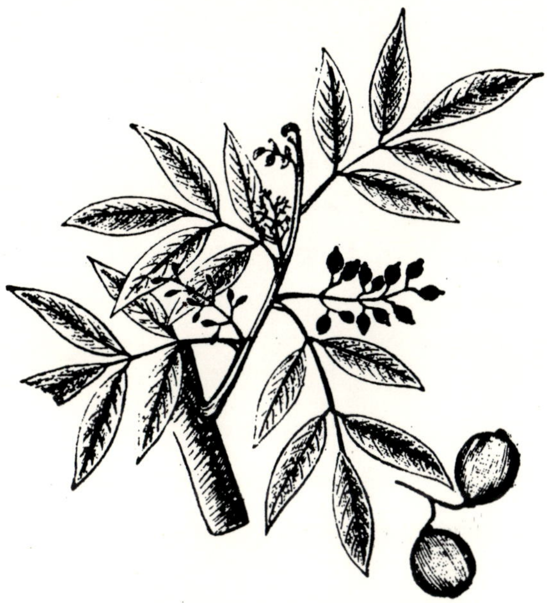

प्रियङ्गोः शाखापत्रफलानि ।

प्रियङ्गुः फलिनी कान्ता लता च महिलाह्वया ।
गुन्द्रा गुन्द्रफला श्यामा विष्वक्सेनाङ्गनाप्रिया ॥
प्रियङ्गुः शीतला तिक्ता तुवरानिलपित्तहृत् ।
रक्ताभियोगदौर्गन्ध्यस्वेददाहज्वरापहा ॥
वान्तिभ्रान्त्यतिसारघ्नी वक्त्रजाड्यविनाशिनी ।
गुल्मतृट्विषमोहघ्नी तद्वद्गन्धप्रियङ्गुका ॥

A specimen page of illustrated Nighaṇṭu, The title page of the early printed edition of the book in Sanskrit *Āyurveda-vijñānam* by Vinod Lal Sengupta, Calcutta.

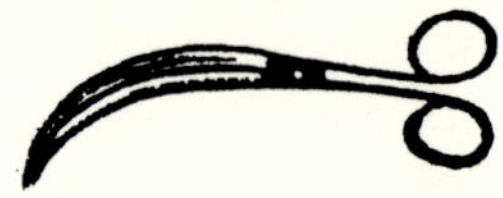

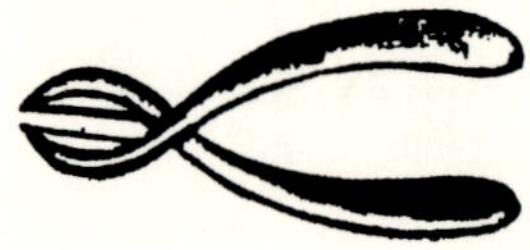

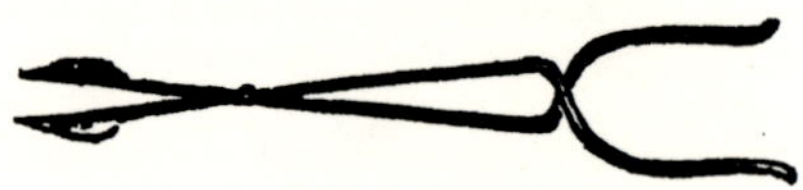

नखशस्त्रम् ।

वक्रर्जुधारं द्विमुखं नखशस्त्रं नवाङ्गुलम् ।
सूक्ष्मशल्योद्धृतिच्छेदभेदप्रच्छानलेखने ॥

दन्तलेखनम् ।

एकधारं चतुष्कोणं प्रबद्धयवाकृति चैकतः ।
दन्तलेखनकं तेन शोधयेद्दन्तशर्करान् ॥

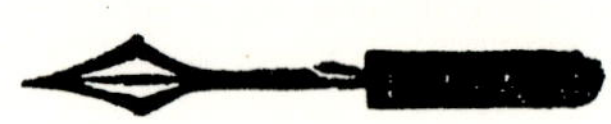

सूची ।

वृत्ता गूढ़दृढ़ाः पाशे तिस्रः सूच्योऽत्र सीवने ।
मांसलानां प्रदेशानां त्र्यस्रा त्र्यङ्गुलमायता ॥
अल्पमांसास्थिसन्धिस्थव्रणानां द्व्यङ्गुलायता ।
व्रीहिवक्त्रा धनुर्वक्रा पक्वामाशयमर्म्मसु ॥
सा सार्द्धत्र्यङ्गुला सर्व्वा वृत्तास्ताः सूचयः स्मृताः ॥

तत्फलं मधुरं रूक्षं कषायं शीतलं गुरु।
विबन्धाध्मानबलकृत् संग्राही कफपित्तजित्॥

अस्यास्त्वचो मात्रा १ माषकः, फलस्य ६ रक्तिकाः।
फलमेवास्याः सदा व्यवह्रियते। प्रियंग, फुलप्रियंग।

कुटजः। (कोरैया। कुठेया। कुड़ा।)

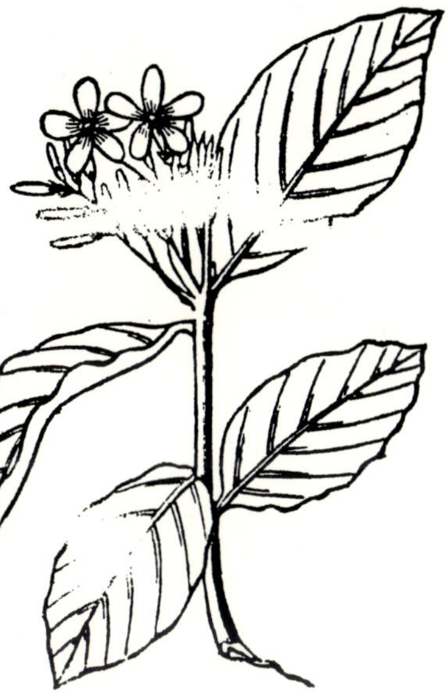

कुटजः कूटजः कौटो वत्सको गिरिमल्लिका।
कालिङ्गः शक्रशाखी च मल्लिकापुष्प इत्यपि।
इन्द्रो यवफलः प्रोक्तो वृक्षकः पाण्डुरद्रुमः॥
कुटजः कटुको रूक्षो दीपनस्तुवरो हिमः।
तिक्तः संग्राहकः प्रोक्तस्त्वग्दोषज्वरनाशनः।

श्रीः ।

वैद्यवरश्रीडल्हणाचार्यविरचितया निबन्धसंग्रहाख्यव्याख्यया

समुल्लसिता

महर्षिणा सुश्रुतेन विरचिता

सुश्रुतसंहिता ।

आयुर्वेदीयग्रन्थमालासंपादकेन

आचार्योपाह्वेन त्रिविक्रमात्मजेन यादवशर्मणा संशोधिता ।

मुम्बय्यां

तुकाराम जावजी

इत्येतैः स्वकीये निर्णयसागरमुद्रायन्त्रालये आयसाक्षरैः

मुद्रापयित्वा प्रसिद्धिं नीता ।

शके १८३७

मूल्यं ८ रूप्यकाः ।

The title-page of *Suśruta-Saṁhitā*, of Nirṇaya-sāgar Press, Bombay.

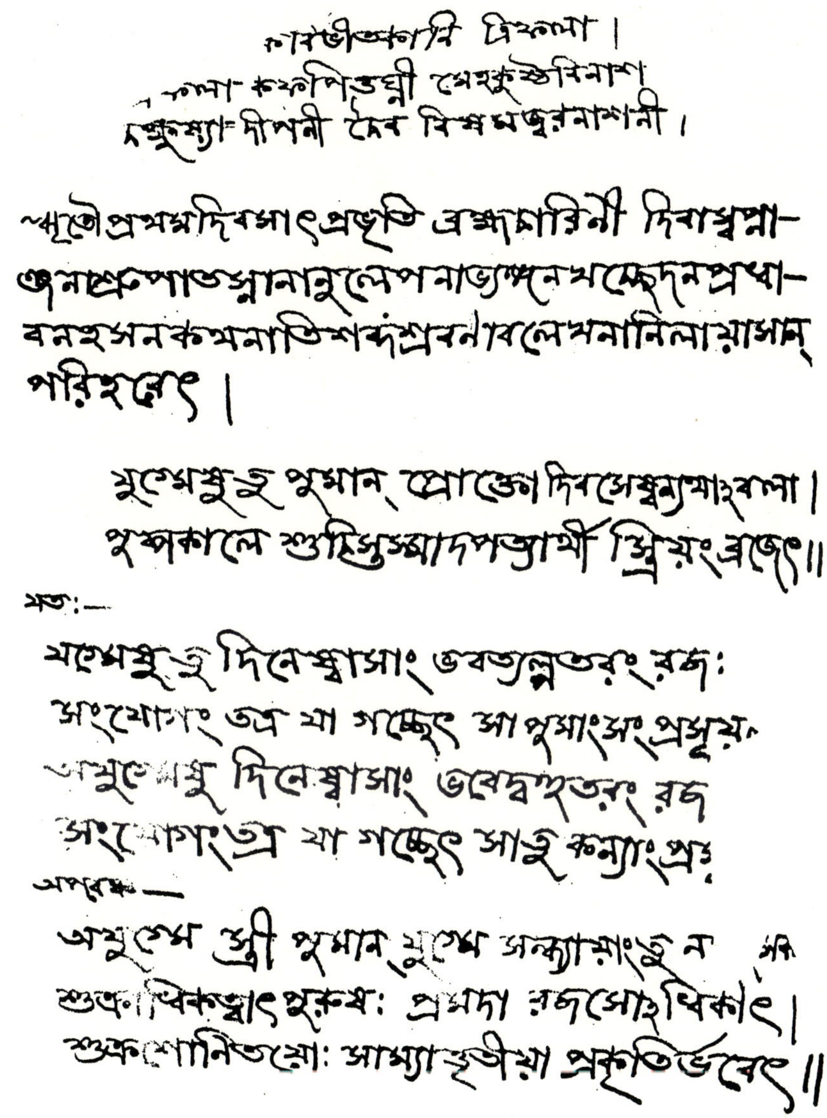

…পাবর্তী… ত্রিফলা।
…কফপিত্তঘ্নী মেহকুষ্ঠবিনাশ
…দীপনী চৈব বিষমজ্বরনাশিনী।

ঋতৌ প্রথমদিবসাৎ প্রভৃতি ব্রহ্মচারিণী দিবাস্বপ্নাঞ্জনাশ্রুপাতস্নানানুলেপনাভ্যঙ্গনখচ্ছেদনপ্রধাবনহসনকথনাতিশব্দশ্রবণাবলেখনানিলায়াসান্ পরিহরেৎ।

যুগ্মেষু তু পুমান্ প্রোক্তো দিবসেষ্বন্যথাঽবলা।
পুষ্পকালে শুচিস্তস্মাদপত্যার্থী স্ত্রিয়ং ব্রজেৎ॥

মত:—

যুগ্মেষু তু দিনেষ্বাসাং ভবত্যল্পতরং রজঃ
সংযোগং তত্র যা গচ্ছেৎ সা পুমাংসং প্রসূয়…
অযুগ্মেষু দিনেষ্বাসাং ভবেদ্বহুতরং রজ
সংযোগং তত্র যা গচ্ছেৎ সা তু কন্যাং প্র…

অপরঞ্চ—

অযুগ্মে স্ত্রী পুমান্ যুগ্মে অন্যাস্বাংতু ন …
শুক্রাধিকত্বাৎ পুরুষঃ প্রমদা রজসোঽধিকাৎ।
শুক্রশোণিতয়োঃ সাম্যাত্তৃতীয়া প্রকৃতির্ভবেৎ॥

A Bengāli physician's Notes on the therapeutics of Suśruta.

पङ्कवट्(टम्) । क्ली । पद्मे । रा.नि.व.१०।

पङ्कवारि । क्ली । काञ्जिके । वै.निघ. ।

पङ्कवासः । पुं । कर्कटे । रा.नि.व.१९ ।

पङ्कशुक्तिः । स्त्री । शम्बी । झिनुक । चिका. ।

पङ्कशू(षू,सू)रणः । पुं। पद्मकन्दे । शालूक । चिका. ।

पङ्कारः । पुं । (Vallisneria, or Tropa bispinosa,) जलजद्रव्यविशेषे, कण्टकसेवल्यां । मे. ।

पङ्किलः । त्रि । पङ्कमये । मलिने ।

पङ्कीरः । पुं । टिट्टिभपक्षिणि । টিটির পাখী । वै.निघ. ।

पङ्केज(रुह)म् । क्ली । कमले । रा.नि.व.१०।

पङ्क्तिकण्टकः । पुं । अपामार्गक्षुपे । रा. नि.व.४ ।

पङ्क्तिकन्दः । मालाकन्दे । रा.नि.व.७।

पङ्क्तिचरः । पुं । कुररपक्षिणि । रा.नि.व. १९ । क्रौञ्चपक्षिणि । श.चि. ।

पङ्क्तिबीजः (कः) । पुं । बर्बूरकवृक्षे । বাবলা গাছ । रा.नि.व.८ । आरग्वधवृक्षे । क- र्णिकारवृक्षे । শোন্দাল, চীনের কদলী গাছ । रा.नि.व.९ ।

पङ्क्तिशूलः । पुं,क्ली । परिणामशूले । निदा- नलक्षणे । "स्वैर्निदानैः प्रकुपितो वातः सन्निहितो यदा । कफपित्ते समावृत्य शूलकारी भवेद्बली । भुक्ते जीर्य्यति यच्छूलं तदेव परिणामजम् । तस्य लक्षणमप्येतत् समासेनाभिधीयते । आध्मानाटोप- विण्मूत्रविबन्धारतिवेपनैः । स्निग्धोष्णोपशमप्रायं वातिकं तद्वदेद्भिषक् । तृष्णादाहारतिस्वेदकट्वम्ल- लवणोत्तमम् । शूलं शीतशमप्रायं पैत्तिकं तद्वदे- द्भिषक् । छर्दिहृल्लाससम्मोहस्वल्परुग्दीर्घसन्ततिः । कटुतिक्तोपशान्ती च विज्ञेयश्च कफात्मकम् ॥" इ- त्यादि । [योर्वधात् ।" सु.नि.१अ. ।

पङ्गुः । पुं । वातव्याधिविशेषे । "पङ्गुः सक्थ्नोः ।

पङ्गुल(ला)हारिणी । स्त्री । शिम्बीक्षुपे ।

पङ्गुत्वम् । क्ली । पङ्गुभावे । रा.नि.व.४ ।

पचनम् । क्ली । पाके । पुं । अग्नौ । श.च. । स्त्री (नी) । वनबीजपूरे । रा.नि.व.११ ।

पचम्पचा । स्त्री । दारुहरिद्रायाम् । प.मु. । भा.म.१भ.तन्द्रिकज्व.चि. । "मरिचकणपचम्पचा- वचारुक् ।"

पचा । स्त्री । पाके । अम. ।

पचेलुकः । पुं । पाचके । चिका. ।

पच्यमानज्वरः । पुं । ज्वरविशेषे । পরিপক্ব জ্বর । लक्षणम्—"ज्वरवेगोऽधिकस्तृष्णा कर्दनो- सारविड्ग्रहाः । मलप्रवृत्तिरुत्क्लेशः पच्यमानस्य लक्षणम् ॥" मा.नि. ।

पञ्चः । पुं । तिक्तपटोले । वै.निघ. ।

पञ्चकट्यम् । क्ली । जीवनपञ्चमूले ह्रस्वपञ्च- मूले च । वा.सू.१५अ. ।

पञ्चकन्दाः । पुं । पञ्चसिद्धौषधिविशेषेषु । ते च तैलकन्दक्षीरकन्दसुधाकन्दरुदन्तीसर्पाक्ष्यात्म- काः । रा.नि.व.२२ । See सिद्धौषधिः ।

पञ्चकपित्थम् । क्ली । कपित्थस्य मूलत्वक्पत्र- फलपुष्पेषु । वा.उ.३८अ. ।

पञ्चकर्म्म । क्ली । वमनविरेकनस्यनिरूहानुवास- नेषु । বমনাদি পাঁচপ্রকার ক্রিয়া । "प्रथमं वमनं पश्चात् विरेकश्चानुवासनं । एतानि पञ्चक- र्म्माणि निरूहो नावनं तथा ॥" भा. । तेषु न्यून- सप्ताब्दे अतीताशीत्यब्दे च नस्यं, ऊनद्वादशे धूमः, ऊनपञ्चमे कवलः, ऊनदशमे अतिक्रान्तसप्ततौ च शोधनं, न्यूनषोडशे सप्ततिवार्षिके च रक्तमोक्षणं न देयम् । एतानि दोषनिर्हरणार्थं यथाकालं प्र- योज्यानि । प.प्र.४ख.। विशेषास्तत्तच्छब्दे लभ्याः ।

पञ्चकषायः । पुं । वचावासापटोलप्रियङ्गुनि- म्बात्मकद्रव्यवर्गे । भा.म.४भ.यो.व्या.चि. । "चूर्णैः पञ्चकषायजैः ।" भैष.कर्परी.चि. ।

पञ्चकोरः । पुं । जलकुक्कुभे । चिका. ।

पञ्चकृत् (त्यः) । पुं । पर्कटीवृक्षे, पक्षीफलवृक्षे। रा.नि.व.८ ।

A specimen page of the Sanskrit medical lexicon prepared by Umesh Chandra Gupta, *Vaidyaka-Śabda Sindhu*, Calcutta.

ಯೋಗರತ್ನಾಕರ

ಎಂಬ

ವೈದ್ಯಗ್ರಂಥ.

ಕರ್ಣಾಟಕಾನ್ಧ್ರಟೀಕಾಸಹಿತ.

YOGARATNÁKARA.

A TREATISE ON MEDICINE COMPILED FROM VARIOUS SOURCES.

TRANSLATED INTO KANNADA AND TELUGU

BY THE

PANDITS OF THE GOVERNMENT ORIENTAL LIBRARY,

MYSORE:

PART I.

Published by the Curator, Government Oriental Library, under the Authority of the Government of His Highness the Maharaja of Mysore.

MYSORE:

PRINTED AT THE GOVERNMENT BRANCH PRESS,

1899.

Prcie Rs 2¼

Title page of *Yoga-ratnākara*, printed in Mysore, in 1899.

36 ಯೋಗರತ್ನಾಕರ—ಅರಿಷ್ಟಲಕ್ಷಣಮ್.

ಮುಂತಾದ) ದೇಹದ್ವಾರಗಳಿಂದಲೂ, ರೋಮಕೂಪೇಭ್ಯಃ—ರೋಮಕೂಪಗಳಿಂದಲೂ, ರಕ್ತಂ ಪ್ರವರ್ತತೇ—ರಕ್ತವು ಹೊರಡುವುದೊ, ಸಃ—ಅವನು, ಸದ್ಯಃ—ಆಗಲೇ, ಜೀವಿತಂ—ಪ್ರಾಣವನ್ನು, ತ್ಯಜೇತ್—ಬಿಡುವನು.

విషముచే కలుగువ్యాధి లేకయుండువానికి రోమకూపములందును నేత్రాది ఇంద్రియద్వారములందును రక్తము ప్రవించిన ఆ నరుడు అప్పుడే మృతిజెందును ॥ ౧౫౭ ॥

सम्यक्चिकित्स्यमानस्य विकारो योऽभिवर्धते ।
प्रक्षीणबलमांसस्य लक्षणं तद्गतायुषः ॥ १५८ ॥

ಸಮ್ಯಕ್—ಚೆನ್ನಾಗಿ (ಶಾಸ್ತ್ರದಲ್ಲಿ ವಿಧಿಸಿರುವಂತೆ), ಚಿಕಿತ್ಸ್ಯಮಾನಸ್ಯ—ಚಿಕಿತ್ಸಿಸಲ್ಪಡುತ್ತಿರುವ ರೋಗಿಗೆ, (ದಿನೇ ದಿನೇ) ಪ್ರಕ್ಷೀಣಬಲಮಾಂಸಸ್ಯ—ಬಲವೂ ಮಾಂಸವೂ ಬಹಳ ಕುಂದಿಹೋಗಿ, ವಿಕಾರೋಽಭಿವರ್ಧತೇ (ಇತಿ) ಯಃ—ರೋಗವು ಹೆಚ್ಚುತ್ತಿರುವುದು ಯಾವದುಂಟೊ, ತತ್—ಅದು, ಗತಾಯುಷಃ—ಆಯುಸ್ಸುಮುಗಿದವನ, ಲಕ್ಷಣಂ—ಚಿಹ್ನೆಯು.

బాగుగ చికిత్సచేయబడుచుండు నరునికి బలిమి మాంసము క్షీణములై, వ్యాధి వృద్ధిజెందిన అది ఆయుస్సు తీరినవానికి లక్షణమని తెలియవలయు ॥ ౧౫౮ ॥

शुष्कास्यः श्यामलोष्ठोऽप्यसितरदततिः शीतनासाप्रदेशः
शोणाक्षश्चैकनेत्रो लुलितकरपदः श्रोत्रपातित्ययुक्तः ।
शीतश्वासोऽथ चोष्णश्वसनसमुदयः शीतगात्रप्रकम्पः
सोद्वेगो निष्प्रपञ्चः प्रभवति मनुजस्सर्वथा मृत्युकाले ॥१५९॥

ಮನುಜಃ—ಮನುಷ್ಯನು, ಮೃತ್ಯುಕಾಲೇ—ಸಾಯುವ ಸಮಯದಲ್ಲಿ, ಶುಷ್ಕಾಸ್ಯಃ—ಬಾಯಾರಿದವನಾಗಿಯೂ, ಶ್ಯಾಮಲೋಷ್ಠಃ—ಕಪ್ಪಾದ ತುಟಿಯುಳ್ಳವನಾಗಿಯೂ, ಅಸಿತರದತತಿಃ—ಕಪ್ಪಾದ ಹಲ್ಲುಸಾಲುಳ್ಳವನಾಗಿಯೂ, ಶೀತನಾಸಾಪ್ರದೇಶಃ—ತಣ್ಣಗಿರುವ ಮೂಗುಳ್ಳವನಾಗಿಯೂ, ಶೋಣಾಕ್ಷಃ—ಕೆಂಪಾದ ಕಣ್ಣುಳ್ಳವನಾಗಿಯೂ, ಏಕನೇತ್ರಃ—ಒಂದೇಕಡೆಯಲ್ಲಿ ದೃಷ್ಟಿಯುಳ್ಳವನಾಗಿಯೂ, ಲುಲಿತಕರಪದಃ—ಕೈಕಾಲುಗಳನ್ನು (ತಿರಿಚುವನಾಗಿಯೂ) ಬೀಸಿ ಹಾಕುವನಾಗಿಯೂ, ಶ್ರೋತ್ರಪಾತಿತ್ಯಯುಕ್ತಃ—ಕಿವಿಜೋಲುಬಿದ್ದವ [ಕಿವುಡ] ನಾಗಿಯೂ, ಶೀತಶ್ವಾಸಃ—ತಣ್ಣಗೆ ಉಸಿರುಬಿಡುವನಾಗಿಯೂ, ಅಥ ಚ—ಒಡನೆಯೇ, ಉಷ್ಣಶ್ವಸನಸಮುದಯಃ—ಬೆಚ್ಚಗೆ ಬೇಗಬೇಗ ಉಸಿರುಬಿಡುವನಾಗಿಯೂ, ಶೀತಗಾತ್ರಪ್ರಕಂಪಃ—ಚಳಿಯಿಂದ ಮೈನಡುಗುವವನಾಗಿಯೂ, ಸೋದ್ವೇಗಃ—ಭಯದಿಂದ ನಡುಗುವವನಾಗಿಯೂ, ನಿಷ್ಪ್ರಪಂಚಃ—ಪ್ರಪಂಚಜ್ಞಾನಶೂನ್ಯನಾಗಿಯೂ, ಸರ್ವಥಾ—ನಾನಾವಿಧವಾಗಿ, ಪ್ರಭವತಿ—ಆಗುವನು.

మరణకాలమునందు నరునికి నోరెండుచును, పెదవి పల్లు నల్లగను, ముక్కు చల్లగను, నేత్రము ఎఱ్ఱనై, రెప్ప వాల్చక చూచుచును, హస్తము పాదము చలించుచును, చెవి జారుపాటుగలిగియు, శ్వాసము కొంతకాలము శీతముగనుండి మరి కొంతకాలము ఉష్ణమగుచును, చలిచే దేహము వణకుచును, భయము కలిగియు, ప్రపంచజ్ఞానము తప్పియు, ఉండును ॥ ॥ ౧౫౯ ॥

अक्षैर्लक्षितलक्षणेन पयसा पूर्णेन्दुना भानुना
पूर्वादक्षिणपश्चिमोत्तरदिशं षट्त्रिद्विमासैककम् ।
छिद्रं पश्यति चेत्तदा दशदिनं धूमाकृतिं पञ्चमे
ज्वालां पश्यति सद्य एव मरणं कालोचितज्ञानिनाम् ॥१६०॥

ಅಕ್ಷೈಃ—ಚಕ್ರಗಳೊಡನೆ, ಪಯಸಾ—ನೀರಿನೊಡನೆ, ಪೂರ್ಣೇಂದುನಾ—ಪೂರ್ಣಚಂದ್ರನೊಡನೆ, ಭಾನುನಾ—ಸೂರ್ಯನೊಡನೆ (ಕೂಡಿರುವಂತೆ), ಪೂರ್ವಾ ದಕ್ಷಿಣಪಶ್ಚಿಮೋತ್ತರ ದಿಶಂ—ಪೂರ್ವದಕ್ಷಿಣಪಶ್ಚಿಮೋತ್ತರದಿಕ್ಕುಗಳನ್ನು, ಪಶ್ಯತಿ ಚೇತ್—ಕಂಡರೆ, (ಕ್ರಮವಾಗಿ) ಷಟ್ತ್ರಿದ್ವಿಮಾಸೈಕಕಂ—ಆರು ಮೂರು ಎರಡು ಒಂದು ಮಾಸಗಳೊಳಗೆ, ಮರಣಂ—ಸಾವು, (ಆಗುವ್ರುದು). ಛಿದ್ರಂ—ರಂಧ್ರವಾಗಿರುವಂತೆ, ಪಶ್ಯತಿ ಚೇತ್—ಕಂಡರೆ, ದಶದಿನಂ—ಹತ್ತುದಿನಗಳೊಳಗೆ, ಮರಣಂ—ಸಾವು, ಧೂಮಾಕೃತಿಂ—ಹೊಗೆಯ ಆಕಾರವನ್ನು, (ಕಂಡರೆ), ಪಂಚಮೇ—ಐದನೆಯದಿವಸದಲ್ಲಿ, (ಮರಣವು). ಜ್ವಾಲಾಂ ಪಶ್ಯತಿ ಚೇತ್—ಉರಿಯನ್ನು ಕಂಡರೆ, ಸದ್ಯ ಏವ—ಆಗಲೇ, ಮರಣಂ—ಸಾವು, (ಎಂದು) ಕಾಲೋಚಿತಜ್ಞಾನಿನಾಂ—ಕಾಲಜ್ಞಾನಿಗಳಿಂದ, ಲಕ್ಷಿತಲಕ್ಷಣೇನ—ನಿರೂಪಿಸಲ್ಪಟ್ಟ ಲಕ್ಷಣದಿಂದ, (ತಿಳಿಯತಕ್ಕದು). ?

పూర్వము దక్షిణము పశ్చిమము ఉత్తరము ఈ దిక్కులయందు క్రమముగ బండిచక్రములు ఉదకము పూర్ణచంద్రుడు సూర్యుడు అగుపడినవారలకు క్రమముగ ఆరు మూడు రెండు ఒకటిమాసములలోపల మరణముగలుగును.

A specimen page of *Yoga-ratnākara*, printed in Mysore in 1899, giving the original Sanskrit text in Kannada characters, and translations in Kannada and Telugu.

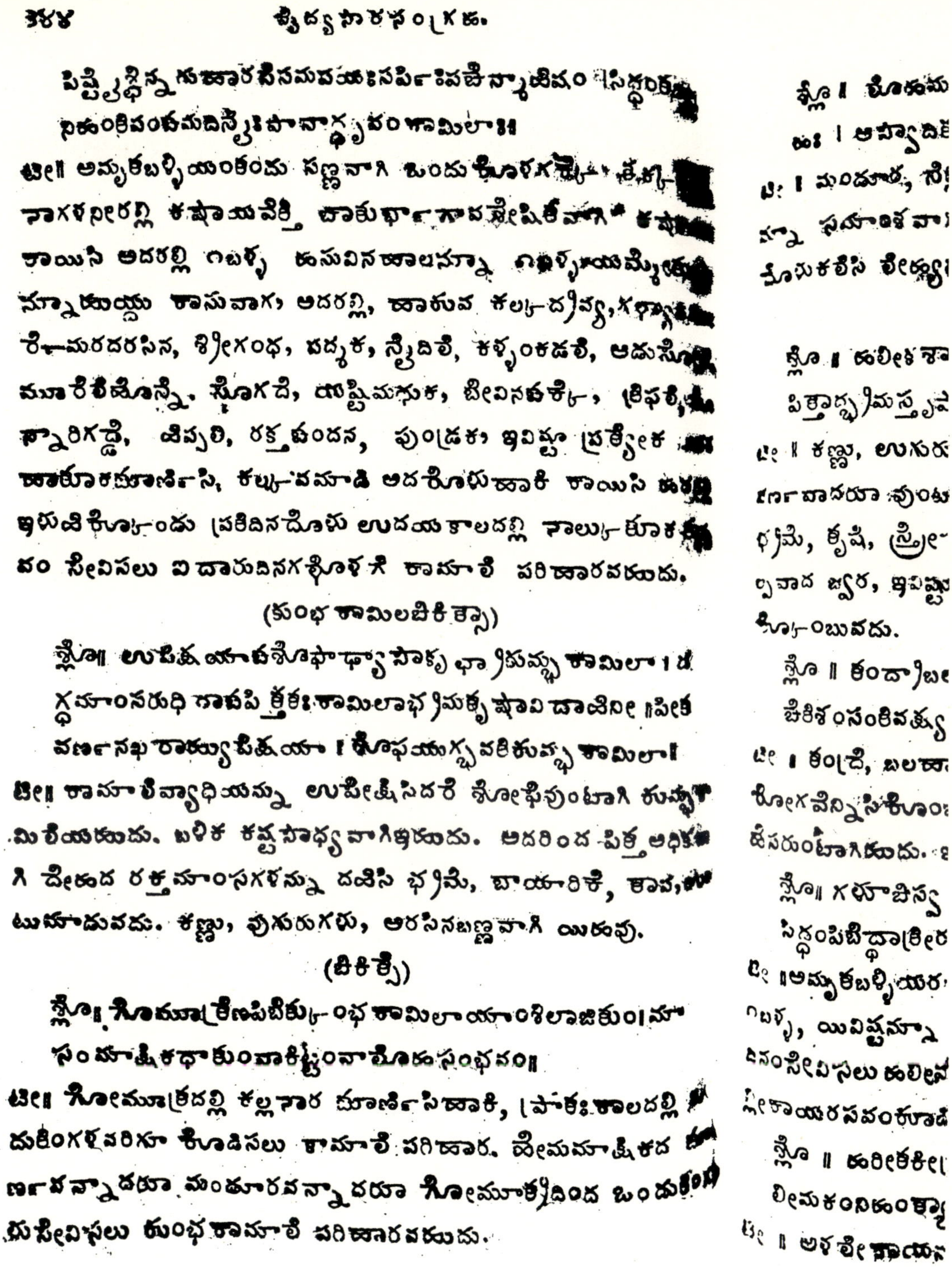
೩೮೪ ವೈದ್ಯಸಾರಸಂಗ್ರಹ.

[illegible]

ಟೀ॥ ಅಮೃತಬಳ್ಳಿಯ ಕಂದು ಸಣ್ಣನಾಗಿ ಒಂದು [illegible] ನಾಗಳನೀರಲ್ಲಿ ಕಷಾಯವಿಕ್ಕಿ [illegible] ಕಾಯಿಸಿ ಅದರಲ್ಲಿ ಗಬಳ್ಳ ಹಸುವಿನಹಾಲನ್ನು [illegible] ನ್ನಾಡುಯ್ದು ಕಾಸುವಾಗ ಅದರಲ್ಲಿ, ಹಾಕುವ ಕಲ್ಕದ್ರವ್ಯ, [illegible] ಕೆಮರದರಸಿನ, ಶ್ರೀಗಂಧ, ಬದ್ಮಕ, ನೈದಿಲೆ, ಕಳ್ಳಂಕಡಲೆ, ಆಡುಸೋ[illegible] ಮೂರೆಲೆಹೊನ್ನೆ, [illegible], ಯಷ್ಟಿಮಧುಕ, ಜೀವಿನಕಕ್ಕೆ, ತ್ರಿಫಳೆ, [illegible] ನ್ನಾರಿಗಡ್ಡೆ, ಹಿಪ್ಪಲಿ, ರಕ್ತಚಂದನ, ಪುಂಡ್ರಕ ಇವಿಷ್ಟು ಪ್ರತ್ಯೇಕ [illegible] ಕಲ್ಕವಮಾಡಿ ಅದರೊಳು ಹಾಕಿ ಕಾಯಿಸಿ [illegible] ಇಳುಹಿಕೊಂಡು ಪ್ರತಿದಿನದೊಳು ಉದಯಕಾಲದಲ್ಲಿ ನಾಲ್ಕುತೊಲ[illegible] ವಂ ಸೇವಿಸಲು ಐದಾರುದಿನಗಳೊಳಗೆ ಕಾಮಾಲೆ ಪರಿಹಾರವಹುದು.

(ಕುಂಭಕಾಮಿಲಚಿಕಿತ್ಸಾ)

ಶ್ಲೋ॥ [illegible]

ಟೀ॥ ಕಾಮಾಲೆವ್ಯಾಧಿಯನ್ನು ಉಪೇಕ್ಷಿಸಿದರೆ ಶೋಫವುಂಟಾಗಿ ಕುಂಭ[illegible] ಮಿಲೆಯಹುದು. ಬಳಿಕ ಕಷ್ಟಸಾಧ್ಯವಾಗಿಹುದು. ಅದರಿಂದ ಪಿತ್ತ ಅಧಿಕ[illegible] ಗಿ ದೇಹದ ರಕ್ತಮಾಂಸಗಳನ್ನು ದಹಿಸಿ ಭ್ರಮೆ, ಬಾಯಾರಿಕೆ, ಕಾವ[illegible] ಟುಮಾಡುವದು. ಕಣ್ಣು, ಉಗುರುಗಳು, ಅರಸಿನಬಣ್ಣವಾಗಿ ಯಿರುವು.

(ಚಿಕಿತ್ಸೆ)

ಶ್ಲೋ॥ ಗೋಮೂತ್ರೇಣಪಿಬೇತ್ಕುಂಭಕಾಮಿಲಾಯಾಂಶಿಲಾಜಿತುಂ॥ ಮಾ[illegible] ಸಂ ಮಾಕ್ಷಿಕಧಾತುಂವಾಕಿಟ್ಟಂವಾಶೋಕಸಂಭವಂ॥

ಟೀ॥ ಗೋಮೂತ್ರದಲ್ಲಿ ಕಲ್ಲನಾರ ದೂಣಿಸಿಹಾಕಿ, ಪ್ರಾತಃಕಾಲದಲ್ಲಿ [illegible] ದುಕಿಂಗಳವರಿಗೂ ಕೊಡಿಸಲು ಕಾಮಾಲೆ ಪರಿಹಾರ. ಹೇಮಮಾಕ್ಷಿಕದ [illegible] ರ್ಣವನ್ನಾದರೂ ಮಂಡೂರವನ್ನಾದರೂ ಗೋಮೂತ್ರದಿಂದ ಒಂದು[illegible] ದುಸೇವಿಸಲು ಕುಂಭಕಾಮಾಲೆ ಪರಿಹಾರವಹುದು.

Page from Vaidya-Sāra-Sangraha, 1882 Bangalore.

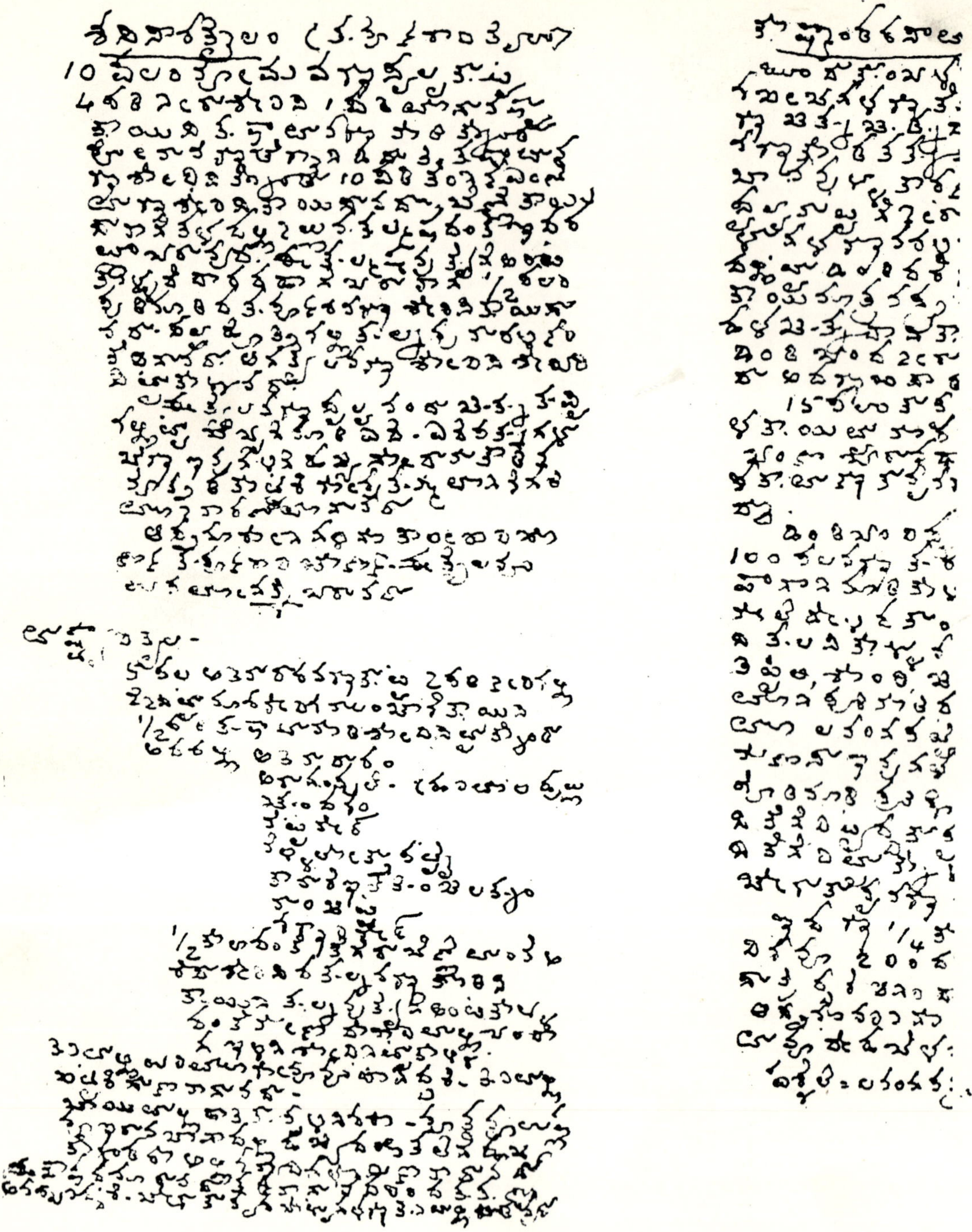

Page from a Physician's note book.